FOREWORD BY
MARSHALL MANDELL, M.D.

ALTERNATIVE HEALTH CARE RESOURCES

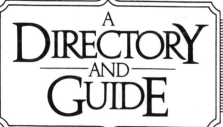

A
DIRECTORY
—AND—
GUIDE

BRETT JASON SINCLAIR

PARKER PUBLISHING COMPANY
West Nyack, New York 10995

Prentice-Hall International, Inc., *London*
Prentice-Hall of Australia, Pty. Ltd., *Sydney*
Prentice-Hall of Canada, Inc., *Toronto*
Prentice-Hall Hispanoamericana, S.A., *Mexico*
Prentice-Hall of India Private Ltd., *New Dehli*
Prentice-Hall of Japan, Inc. *Tokyo*
Prentice-Hall of Southeast Asia Pte., Ltd., *Singapore*
Editora Prentice-Hall do Brasil Ltda., *Rio de Janeiro*

© 1992 by
Brett Jason Sinclair.

10 9 8 7 6 5 4 3 2 1

Library of Congress Cataloging-in-Publication Data

Sinclair, Brett Jason.
    Alternative health care resources : a directory and
guide / Brett Jason Sinclair.
        p.   cm.
    Includes index.
    ISBN 0-13-156522-2   ISBN 0-13-030073-X
    1. Alternative medicine—United States—Directories.
    2. Alternative medicine—Information services—United
States—Directories.   I. Title.
R733.S56 1992   92-28096
362.1'025'73—dc20   CIP

ISBN 0-13-030073-X NB2I

ISBN 0-13-156522-2 PBK

Parker Publishing Company
Business Information & Publishing Division
West Nyack, NY 10995
Simon & Schuster, A Paramount Communications Company

FOREWORD

Modern medicine has often overlooked, ignored, or rejected effective treatments, modern and ancient, which can do much to alleviate the suffering of many forms of physical and mental illness that affect millions of children and adults throughout the world.

Each individual, spouse, parent, or other responsible person has the right to be fully informed about these therapeutic advances: their advantages and disadvantages. With *Alternative Health Care Resources*, a comprehensive volume containing nearly 400 resources, readers are finally in a position to review numerous innovative approaches to the illnesses they are concerned about; make an intelligent choice among them; and advise their physicians as to how they wish to have their health problems managed.

If a far-ranging, open-minded, and respectfully conducted discussion does not lead to a meeting of the minds between attending physician and patient (or those deeply concerned about the patient's welfare), this book will be invaluable. It gives the decision maker(s) the means to contact unlimited health resources—otherwise unknown to them—from whom they can obtain additional information and help.

Alternative Health Care Resources enables readers to select members of the healing profession whose philosophies and methods of treatment are in harmony with their wishes. This, in turn, creates a highly desirable atmosphere of caring cooperation in which to carry out mutually agreed-upon overall case management.

Decision making by an intelligent and informed person can be a very difficult process. Most people have no background in many of the complex areas often involved in the diagnostic approaches and methods of care of a serious illness. In the ever-evolving field of human health sciences, there are many possibilities and no guarantees that a given approach will be effective in all cases of a particular disorder.

Making what one believes to be the best choice among several attractive and reasonable choices can be a nerve-wracking and time-consuming responsibility beset with frustration and honest doubt. It may be necessary to try a series of promising options before finding the solution to a complex medical problem. My advice, should you find yourself in this difficult situation, is to do your "honest best" to keep on top of things and seek expert advice as needed during the course of the illness. *Alternative Health Care Resources* will help guide you to appropriate sources of information.

Brett Sinclair, the author of *Alternative Health Care Resources* has carefully and objectively evaluated the various services offered for the reader's consideration. He has personally contacted and "exhaustively researched every resource, making certain that each met his rigorous standards of providing the most up-to-date and accurate information." He tells me he has deliberately excluded "personal judgments or opinions about treatments and lifestyles" and, instead, provides his readers with "an objective array of options" and does no "advertising." His objective in writing *Alternative Health Care Resources* is "to empower readers with the knowledge that they need to develop confidence in their own judgment and native intelligence: seeking truth objectively rather than emotionally, and not, by blind proxy, uncritically relinquishing their health or the health of loved ones to dogmatic assumptions of modern medical practice."

Knowing that you have a choice about the nature of the health care you or someone you care about will receive, is a serious obligation. It is necessary for you to carefully review the treatments and claims made for them. Be aware. Be objective. Be critical. Ask questions. Having a choice carries with it a heavy responsibility, but being in the fortunate position of having a choice means that this option can be exercised with great care.

Marshall Mandell, M.D.

ABOUT THIS BOOK

The *Annals of Internal Medicine* (no. 101, July 1984, pp. 105–112) described a University of Pennsylvania study in which researchers found that the higher a person's education level, the more likely he or she would be to choose alternative health care treatment. The study's numbers are telling: 40% of all those who have attended college would choose alternative care over conventional. The conclusions of a study presented in the *American Journal of Epidemiology* (no. 127, February 1988, pp. 297–309) echo the same statistics with respect to vitamin supplements: The better educated you are, the more likely you are to take supplemental nutrients.

But even in this age of information glut, accurate and reliable information on alternative approaches to degenerative diseases, chronic conditions, and the lifestyle changes that can help prevent them is often hard to come by. Unless you *happen* to know someone who has undergone an alternative treatment or you *accidentally* stumble over the information, it may be nearly impossible to find. A health care professional experienced in alternative therapies may be even more difficult to locate.

Alternative Health Care Resources: A Directory and Guide answers the need for more readily available information on all aspects of alternative health care. It is a comprehensive guide to almost 400 self-help groups, professional organizations, institutions, foundations, journals, magazines, and newsletters that provide information on alternative treatments, disease-preventive lifestyle changes, and health-related issues.

This book is organized alphabetically by health condition or health-related topic, and it covers a range of subjects including AIDS, allergies, antibiotics, circumcision, environmental illness, nutrition and diet, osteoporosis, pain relief, and pesticides. For each topic covered, you will find listings of all the major organizations and publications that offer assistance and information. The resources under each subject heading include:

Self-Help Groups. These groups are made up of people who have had chronic or acute conditions or degenerative diseases and who have benefited from alternative treatments. In addition to providing information about a specific condition or disease, these groups will give you emotional support and will often recommend physicians and other health professionals if needed.

Organizations of Professional Health Care Providers. These organizations will provide you with guidance and information on natural therapies as well as referrals to classically trained physicians or other licensed and accredited practitioners.

Scientific Journals, Popular Lay Magazines, and Newsletters. These publications offer information on the latest health and medical breakthroughs as well as centuries-old, time-tested folk remedies from around the world.

Institutions and Foundations. These groups offer a variety of viewpoints on such diverse topics as natural childbirth and midwifery, organically grown foods, nutrition and diet, stress-reduction techniques, acupuncture, homeopathy, chronic pain relief, herbal medicine, guided imagery, exercise, longevity, and even holistic dental care.

Provided for each of these resources are:

- complete name and address; telephone number and fax number if available
- toll-free telephone number if available
- contact person if available
- detailed background information on the organization or publication
- up-to-date information on all the services offered
- what you can expect when you contact each resource.

In many cases, assistance and information is free or provided for a small donation.

All the information included in this book was obtained firsthand. I personally contacted each and every listing to ensure that the information was *up-to-date, accurate,* and *complete. Organizations that would not cooperate or that I could not contact personally were not included in the book.* In addition, I studied at least six issues of each journal, magazine, or newsletter to see exactly what kind of information each publication offers.

This information includes some of the best-documented and tested, most benign and reasonable ideas on better health through alternative approaches. Much of this information appears neither in the mass media nor in physicians' journals. Often it must be around for a generation or two before it becomes accepted by traditional medical establishment and before the general public can benefit from it. It is information that could help save your life: therapies for diseases that kill, cripple, or debilitate and preventive techniques that could dramatically cut down your odds of getting these diseases and myriad other health conditions.

One caution: Do not look to this information as polemics against chemotherapy, pharmaceuticals, triple bypass surgery, and medical orthodoxy. Nor should you expect a hosanna to the virtues of vegetarianism, megavitamins, herbs, meditation, and alternative healing. *Rather, this book is strictly an information resource,* a complete guide to finding the right organization to contact for information on particular health conditions, alternative health care treatments and health-related issues.

HOW TO USE THIS BOOK

Alternative Health Care Resources: A Directory and Guide has been specially designed for easy use. Following are some of the features that will enable you to find the information you need quickly and easily.

- The book is organized alphabetically by subject heading, and the contents provides an A–Z listing of each topic covered in the book.
- The resources provided for each topic are also listed alphabetically.
- A detailed index lists each of the almost 400 resources included in the book as well as each subject heading.
- Since many resources offer help and information on a variety of topics, you will find extensive cross-referencing throughout the book. After the last resource listing under a topic heading, you will find the names of other resources in the book that may also be useful.

CONTENTS

AIDS 1
Allergies 5
Alternative Healing 10
Alzheimer's Disease 24
Amytrophic Lateral Sclerosis 27
Antibiotics 29
Aromatherapy 31
Arthritis and Other Rheumatoid Diseases 35
Asthma 37
Autism 40
Ayurvedic Medicine 44
Bee Venom Therapy 46
Biomagnetics 47
Cancer 51
Candida Albicans 66
Chelation Therapy 68
Childbirth 71
Childhood Ailments 88
Chronic Fatigue Syndrome 99
Circumcision 102
Colitis and Crohn's Disease 103
Colon Therapy 104
Color Therapy 106
Computer Database Searching 107
Crystal Healing 109
Dental Health 110
Dyslexia and Scoptopic Sensitivity Syndrome 115
Eating Disorders 118
Endometriosis 124
Environmental Illness 126
Epilepsy 140

Eye Disorders 142
Fitness 147
Flower Essence Remedies 150
Food Allergies 152
Food Irradiation 157
Handicapped 160
Headaches 162
Head Injuries 165
Healing Centers 167
Health Self-Education 169
Hearing Problems 176
Heart Disease, High Blood Pressure, and Stroke 178
Herbalism 184
Herpes 192
Homeopathy 194
Hospice 200
Hypnotherapy 202
Hypoglycemia 208
Imagery 211
Incontinence 214
Iridology 217
Lifestyle 219
Longevity and Aging 228
Lupus Erythematosis 237
Medical Consumerism 239
Medical/Health Care Fraud 244
Medical/Health Care Freedom of Choice 246
Medical/Health Care Rights 255
Mind-Body Connection 258
Muscle Testing and Diagnosis 279
Natural Hygiene 285
Naturopathy 290
Neurofibromatosis 293
Nutrition and Diet 295
Obsessive-Compulsive Disorders 319
Organic Food 322
Oriental Healing and Exercise 328
Orthomolecular Nutrition and Therapy 342
Osteoporosis 347

Oxidative Therapies   349
Pain Relief   353
Parenting   373
Parkinson's Disease   379
Pesticides   381
Prevention   386
Psoriasis   419
Psychological Healing   421
Rare Diseases   442
Respiratory Illnesses   444
Scleroderma   446
Seasonal Affective Disorder   447
Sjögren's Syndrome   450
Speech Problems   452
Sports Medicine   457
Stress Reduction   459
Substance Abuse   463
Support Groups   466
Temporomandibular Joint Disease   471
Tinnitus   473
Tourette Syndrome   474
Traveling Abroad   476
Veterinary Health Care   477
Water Fluoridation   479
Weight Loss   481
Women's Health Issues   482

Index   489

A PERSONAL NOTE

Not unexpectedly, with close to 400 organizations and publications listed, differing—even conflicting—opinions exist between them. With such myriad alternative, holistic, and complementary therapies and viewpoints on lifestyle changes, it is inevitable that you will disagree with the findings and conclusions of some and be unimpressed by others. However, some will convince you and will prove quite valuable. But it is not for me, or indeed for anyone else, to say which therapy or lifestyle change is best for you. You must choose for yourself from all that is available, alternative as well as conventional. No ratings of any group or publication is included in this book. Rather than accept the opinions of so-called experts on the value of alternative health care, which treatment is best, and what diet and lifestyle change will prove most effective, I hope you will carefully look at the information provided to you by these resources—as well as what traditional medicine can offer—and then judge for yourself what makes the most sense for your particular needs. If you do that, then this book's purpose—*to offer you a real choice*— will be well served.

Brett Jason Sinclair

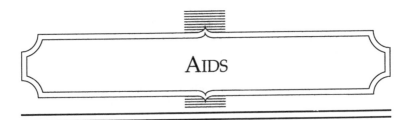

AIDS

AIDS Treatment News
P.O. Box 411256
San Francisco, CA 94141
415-255-0588
415-255-4659 (fax)

Contact: John S. James

▌Background

In spite of medical orthodoxy's reassurances that AZT is the only treatment available for acquired immune deficiency syndrome (AIDS), many physicians and scientists from around the world believe otherwise.

AIDS Treatment News, a six- to eight-page, biweekly newsletter ($30 for AIDS or AIDS-related complex, ARC patients, $100 for nonprofit institutions, $200 for businesses—24 issues), reports on new HIV and AIDS treatments as well as on public policy matters.

▌What's Offered

AIDS Treatment News focuses solely on experimental and complementary therapies. Rather than treatments that are in an experimental stage, it concentrates on those therapies that are available now. All information is collected from medical journals, interviews with scientists and physicians, and AIDS or ARC patients.

All back issues may be ordered in a group or individually. Some specific therapies explored in depth and over several issues include the uses of DDI, compound Q, fluconazole, AZT, aerosol

1

pentamidine, ganciclovir (DHPG), diclazuril, DHEA, lentinan, peptide T, passive immunotherapy, and hypericin.

Totally eclectic, this newsletter concerns itself only with what has shown promise, no matter what the source or where the information comes from. Articles are usually no more than a page or two, always give references, and usually have case histories when available. Examples of treatments and other AIDS-related issues covered in recent issues are:

- Blue-green algae antiviral compounds
- Interferon and Kaposi's sarcoma
- Hypericin survey
- World AIDS Day
- Flu shots for HIV-positive individuals
- AZT dosages
- Cryptosporidiosis.

Telephone, fax, or write for a sample issue.

Foundation for Research of Natural Therapies
Human Energy Press
1020 Foster City
Suite 205
Foster City, CA 94404
415-349-0718
415-349-1257 (fax)

▌ Background

The Foundation for Research of Natural Therapies sponsors conferences, publishes, and sells audio tapes and videos exploring a variety of nontoxic, drugless, alternative, or complementary treatments for chronic degenerative diseases.

▌ What's Offered

Much of the available information is on AIDS. However, since many of the therapies discussed bolster and stimulate the immune system, they may prove to be of benefit to everyone. Literally hundreds of audio cassettes and dozens of videos from around the world are available. All were prepared by, and feature, the physician or scientist who has developed and uses the therapy. Examples of some of the videos are:

▮ Compound Q (use of the cucumber extract is presented by San Francisco–based Dr. Larry Waites)
▮ Ascorbate (megadoses of intravenous vitamin C is presented by Dr. Robert Cathcart)
▮ Thymic hormones (immunotherapy with thymus extract from Germany is presented by Dr. Milan Pesic).

Audio tapes also run the gamut of treatments and include:

▮ Vitamins and minerals (Peter Duesberg, Ph.D.)
▮ Ozone therapy (Dr. Horst Kief)
▮ Nigelia Sativa (Osama Kandi, Ph.D.)
▮ Fungal extracts (Dr. Erik Enby)
▮ Electromagnetic therapy (G. Rein, Ph.D., et al.).

Audios are $8 each and videos are between $28 (45 minutes) and $160 (five hours).

Health Education AIDS Liaison
HEAL
P.O. Box 1103
Old Chelsea Station
New York, NY 10113
212-674-HOPE

▌ Background

In spite of official pronouncements from the orthodox medical community and the federal government, many people (including reputable scientists from all over the world) believe that therapies other than AZT, such as diet, nutritional supplementation, botanical medicine, and newly discovered pharmaceuticals derived from plants, can benefit AIDS patients.

The Health Education AIDS Liaison (HEAL) was organized to support AIDS patients and to provide information on the use of natural ways of healing through alternative, nontoxic therapies.

▌ What's Offered

HEAL's four-page, quarterly newsletter provides detailed information on both the benefits of alternative treatments and the toxicity found in the treatment of choice in the United States: AZT. HEAL also makes available several information packets on natural therapies, the immune system, and other modalities for treating AIDS.

HEAL is solely supported by contributions from the sale of these items.

Further Resources
Arlin J. Brown Information Center, Inc.
Linus Pauling Institute of Science and Medicine

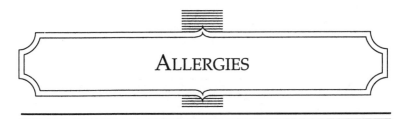

ALLERGIES

Allergic Athlete's Handbook
Official Chlor-Trimeton Handbook for the Allergic Athlete
P.O. Box 5129
Department HV
Bergenfield, NJ 07621

▌Background

If you are one of the 40 million Americans who sneeze and sniffle in late summer and fall, the chances are that you are a hay fever sufferer—allergic to ragweed and pollen. If that's making you throw in the towel every time someone wants to engage in outdoor athletics at that time, then prepare yourself to get instant relief.

The *Allergic Athlete's Handbook* was designed to help hay fever sufferers maintain an active, outdoor life even in the midst of a high pollen count.

▌What's Offered

This free book will provide both the regular or weekend athlete with:

▪ Tips to minimize your exposure to seasonal allergies while you continue to exercise and engage in outdoor sports
▪ A list of recommended sports and other outdoor activities to engage in for allergy sufferers
▪ A national, region-by-region look at seasonal allergies and their peak periods.

To get this helpful book, send a business-sized, self-addressed, stamped envelope.

Allergy Information Association
65 Tromley Drive
Suite 10
Etabicoke
Ontario, Canada M9B 5Y7
416-244-8585
416-234-0777 (fax)

Contact: Brenda Gadbois, Executive Assistant

Background

Allergies take their toll on millions of people every year. Hay fever and asthma rank first in prevalence among all chronic diseases. While it is possible to find a grass-roots organization devoted to a single allergen, finding one that disseminates alternative information on all allergies is quite difficult.

The Allergy Information Association represents not health care professionals but allergy sufferers. Its purpose is to increase the control allergy sufferers have over their own lives by providing:

- Information about allergens
- Education for the general public and the health care community
- Advocacy for ingredient labeling laws and nonorthodox approaches.

What's Offered

Membership ($25) entitles you to a subscription to the 26-page paperback-book sized *Allergy Quarterly*. Regular features include readers' letters, book reviews, product information, environmental concerns, answers to readers' queries, and organization news. Articles are short and newsy and are written by an editorial staff of professionals. Recent topics discussed are:

I Anaphylactic food reactions in children
I Milk allergies in babies
I Asthma education
I Dental fillings
I Hazards of homemade chemicals.

Dozens of booklets on different allergies from additives to sulfite reactions, several cookbooks, and a list of recommended reading material are also available.

American Academy of Environmental Medicine
P.O. Box 16106
Denver, CO 80216
303-622-9755

I **Background**

Have you ever started to sneeze with no apparent reason and then just as suddenly stopped? Have you ever felt that you just had to sleep after eating a particular food? Have you ever smelled something that made you dizzy, nauseous, or weak? If so, something—that you ate, drank, or breathed in—has affected you.

The branch of medicine that may help you when orthodox allergists fail is called environmental medicine.

The American Academy of Environmental Medicine is the professional organization of the several hundred physicians devoted to the practice of environmental medicine. Its members, all physicians themselves, help patients uncover the cause-and-effect relationship between their environment and their illnesses.

▎ What's Offered

Without going into detail, treatment consists of a detailed environmentally oriented history and a series of tests to determine if you are allergic to anything, and if so, what. Treatment may be total avoidance, environmental control, such as air filters or rotational diet, and optimal-dose immunization therapy (to control adverse responses and to increase tolerances for unavoidable allergens).

The Academy has dozens of books on allergies, nutrition, and cooking for allergy sufferers that you may purchase.

If you wish a referral to an environmental medicine specialist (also known as a clinical ecologist) in your area, please send $1 and a self-addressed, stamped envelope.

Pan American Allergy Society
P.O. Box 947
Fredericksburg, TX 78624
512-997-9853

▎ Background

Many people are allergic to something in their environment. Some are born with the allergy; others develop allergic reactions only after repeated exposures. It is often very difficult for a physician to find the allergen.

The Pan American Allergy Society (PAAS) serves as a training group for health care practitioners engaged in the diagnosis and treatment of allergic disorders.

▎ What's Offered

PAAS provides education and training to professionals in the areas of:

I Inhalant, food, and viral allergens
I Immunology
I Allergen testing.

PAAS' training is not in the study of allergies but in showing the connection between aging and the environment on people suffering from allergies and what the professional can do to help. While membership is not available to interested lay individuals, one of PAAS' members practicing in your area may help you if you believe that an allergen is the cause of your ailment.

Further Resources
Enviro-Tech Products
Practical Allergy Research Foundation
Touch For Health Foundation

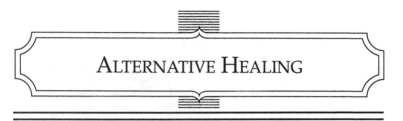

ALTERNATIVE HEALING

Alliance/Foundation for Alternative Medicine
P.O. Box 59
Liberty Lake, WA 99019
509-255-9246

Contact: Marge Jacob

▋ Background

The goals of the Alliance for Alternative Medicine (AAM) and its
sister organization, the Foundation for Alternative Medicine, are
to do more than preserve our shrinking medical freedom of choice.
Those goals are:

- ▋ To encourage legislature that will assure it and to pursue
  education for the general public that will allow it to prosper
- ▋ To develop a cost-effective methodology to evaluate alternative therapies
- ▋ To collect clinical data on the effectiveness of alternative
  medicine.

▋ What's Offered

The Alliance maintains a worldwide network of political advocates
promoting the cause of alternative therapies in their respective
countries. This allows the free flow of information on successful
political strategies.

The Foundation offers material on current research in alternative health care and disease prevention through a list of publications and resources. These resources include books listing

alternative health care practitioners and reports on current findings and practical advice.

AAM's eight-page, quarterly newsletter, *New Horizons*, keeps members informed of current legislative activities and clinical advances in alternative therapies.

American Holistic Medical Association
2002 Eastlake Avenue East
Seattle, WA 98102
206-322-6842

Contact: Suzan Walter

▌ Background

What is holistic medicine? Rather than after-the-fact intervention and treatments almost exclusively involving prescription drugs and surgery intervention, holisic health care focuses on:

▌ Personal responsibility for your own health
▌ Prevention through lifestyle changes, nutrient supplementation, diet, and exercise
▌ Safe nontoxic medical prescriptions and intervention when needed.

The American Holistic Medical Association (AHMA) is a professional organization of holistic health care practitioners, professional and nonprofessional, health-related organizations, businesses, and interested individuals. The AHMA supports research and educational projects that promote holistic medicine.

❚ What's Offered

A nonprofessional general membership ($25) entitles you to the Association's bimonthly, 30-page *Holistic Medicine*. Article topics are directed towards the professional and consist primarily of clinical case studies, in-depth prevention and treatment articles, book reviews, healthy living resources and programs, and AHMA news and a schedule of upcoming events.

Nutritional and fitness guidelines, along with a directory of members (to help you find a physician in your area), are also published and available for sale.

The AHMA will be happy to answer any questions about holistic medicine and will provide a referral to a holistic physician in your area.

American Holistic Nurses' Association
4101 Lake Boone Trail
Suite 201
Raleigh, NC 27607
919-787-5181

❚ Background

In a serious illness, even during a thorough medical examination, a physician is only part of the health care team. A nurse is often part of that team. In many instances, the nurse may be the person spending the most time caring for the patient.

The American Holistic Nurses' Association (AHNA) is a professional organization of nurses who believe that the major purpose of nursing is to assist other professionals toward the health of the patient. The Association defines health as the harmonious balance of mind, body, and spirit, not the relief of symptoms defined in a medical textbook.

▌ What's Offered

Membership in AHNA is only open to professional nurses. A monthly ($16) magazine, *Beginnings*, is available to anyone and contains news of holistic nursing, a calendar of upcoming events, and timely news of the organization. The AHNA maintains and supports the networking of its members in a region or state and will help you to locate a holistic-oriented nurse in your community.

American Raum & Zeit
P.O. Box 1508
Mount Vernon, WA 98273
206-424-6034
206-424-6029 (fax)

▌ Background

Few Americans feel comfortable with science. The writing is obtuse, the vocabulary deliberately arcane, and the conclusions often obscure. When that science is leading-edge the problem is made worse—is it even believable? Yet, the information may prove of such value that the struggle and the suspension of disbelief proves worthwhile.

American Raum & Zeit calls itself the "New Dimension in Scientific Research" and is the American counterpart to a German journal of new and leading-edge science with the same name.

▌ What's Offered

Far more than alternative health care can be found in each 80-odd-page, bimonthly ($59) edition of *Raum & Zeit*. Articles cover all aspects of extraordinary science including physics, electrical energy, book reviews, and a calendar of upcoming events.

Every article is written by a recognized international authority (many articles are translations of material from foreign publications usually unavailable in the United States). Articles are scholarly and, regrettably, not entirely free from technical jargon; nevertheless anyone willing to spend the time and take the effort will find the information understandable. Numerous references from respected journals and scholarly books are at each article's end and will serve the reader for follow-up research. Rather than describe the type of articles on alternative health care you will find, here is a list of recent article topics that relate to alternative health care:

- Contaminated water
- Effects of light and color on physiology
- Fats, oils, and fatty acids and human health
- Ionizing oxygen
- Carpal tunnel syndrome
- Garlic and breast cancer
- Magnets and drinking water
- Natural approach to malignant tumor treatment
- Antioxidant nutrients
- Noninvasive medicine
- Magnetism and youth.

Association of Health Practitioners
P.O. Box 5007
Durango, CO 81301
303-259-1091

Background

Trade or professional associations are formed to benefit their members. They can also benefit the public through education to their members and the public and by providing standards of practice and referrals to their members.

The Association of Health Practitioners is a professional organization of (primarily) dentists and physicians who provide alternative therapies and oppose the use of all toxic materials or materials that have the potential of being toxic.

▌ What's Offered

While the Association is relatively new, it hopes to soon publish a magazine of alternative health care to the general public and a peer-review journal to its members.

At the time of this book's publication you may write or telephone for referrals to members in your area.

Bio-Research For Global Evolution
P.O. Box 3427
Eugene, OR 97403
503-345-9855

▌ Background

I, for one, do not like to read about some topic in alternative healing (or much else for that matter) without seeing the scientific basis on which it is based. Although quite a few information sources have references and citations, very few of these sources use them as more than a hook on which to hang their information. Scientific foundations are not often used to reach new conclusions, conclusions that prove of immediate practical value.

Bio-Research For Global Evolution's four-page, monthly ($20) newsletter, the work of Ray Peat, Ph.D., does just that with special emphasis on nutrition, natural approaches to diseases, regenerative therapies, and antistress methodologies.

▌ What's Offered

Each issue is devoted to a single topic, usually a general one. However, every sentence, every paragraph will either fill you in with the necessary background information to understand the topic or discuss a specific benefit to be derived from adapting to a lifestyle change, using a nutrient, or undertaking a preventive health measure.

The reading is not for the faint-hearted or the mildly interested; you will have to make an effort to grasp fully all that is said and then decide what action to take (if any) to use its conclusions. Recent topics covered have been:

▌ Adaptogens—substances to boost the immune system
▌ Stress and the heart
▌ Nutrition and women
▌ Brain research in Russia.

Back issues of the newsletter, article reprints, and Peat's books are also available.

Health World
Health World, Inc.
1477 Rollins Road
Burlingame, CA 94010
415-343-1637
415-343-0503 (fax)

▌ Background

A full-color bimonthly ($10.50), *Health World* focuses its attention on providing advice on health from an alternative perspective. Information ranges from vitamins, nutrition, health foods, chiropractic care, and homeopathy to traditional Chinese medicine.

▌ What's Offered

Articles cover many areas of health and disease prevention but primarily concern themselves with alternative treatments for diseases and common maladies. Regular monthly columns provide two- to three-paragraph summaries of currently available information on book, music, and video reviews; nutrition and chiropractic news; current medical research; and sports and fitness. All articles are quite scholarly but free from jargon and terminology. Most articles are written by professional practitioners and scientists rather than by journalists. Research papers and scholars are often cited. Practical advice and the pros and cons of a treatment, herb, or nutrient are also discussed. Recent article topics have included:

▐ Epstein-Barr virus—homeopathic medicines
▐ Therapeutic benefits of Di-methylsulfoxide (DMSO)
▐ Saw palmetto—benefits to the immune system
▐ Oxygen—therapeutic benefits
▐ Chromium picolinate—cholesterol balancing
▐ Children's allergies—megavitamin treatment
▐ Homeopathy
▐ Immune system
▐ Nutrition and surgery.

International Society for the Study of Subtle Energies and Energy Medicine
356 Goldco Circle
Golden, CO 80401
303-278-2228
Contact: C. Penny Hiernu, Executive Director

▌ Background

We live in an ocean of energy. We, aside from a physical body, are our own ocean of energy. How do these two oceans act and interact with each other? Does this enhance or perturb health?

The International Society for the Study of Subtle Energies and Energy Medicine was formed to study these energies and their interaction with the human psyche and physiology.

▮ What's Offered

Although primarily made up of scientists and health care practitioners, membership is open to anyone and includes a subscription to the Society's quarterly journal, *Subtle Energies and Medicine*. Technical and directed toward the scientifically literate (and trained), each article topic is more fascinating than the rest. More theoretical than practical (although often enough material is covered to make practical application feasible), every article is replete with references and citations. Recent issue topics were:

- Noncontact therapeutic touch—effect on wound healing rates
- Psychophysiological self-regulation—human potential
- Geomagnetic activity—effect upon cognition
- Shamanistic healing—physiological aspects
- Geomagnetic activity—effect upon violent crime
- Clinical approach to autistic recovery.

Conference proceedings are available as well as a quarterly newsletter that discusses (in less technical detail than the journal) numerous aspects of energy medicine such as psi healing, healer methods, field and energy research instrumentation, and new age science. It also includes readers' letters and comments, book reviews, and interviews.

Journal of Alternative and Complementary Medicine
Argus Health Publications
Manner House
53A High Street
Bag Shot, Surrey
GU 19 5AH, U.K.
0235-353535

Contact: Richard Thomas, Editor

▌Background

Many Americans are surprised to learn that herbal preparations outsell over-the-counter pharmaceuticals throughout Europe. In many cases they are the treatment of choice and are preferred over prescription drugs in numerous countries throughout the world.

Despite this, there are but a few sources of information for the general public on alternative therapies and differing viewpoints on the causes of both common maladies and chronic diseases available outside the United States.

The monthly *Journal of Alternative and Complementary Medicine* (*JACM*) is the premier English publication exclusively devoted to alternative and complementary medicine written for health care professionals and interested individuals.

▌What's Offered

JACM is available in the United States only through subscription from its U.K. publishers. To those Americans who are Anglophiles, the writing in this publication will sound much like an episode from "Upstairs Downstairs"—literate, witty, and charming are but a few of the adjectives that describe *JACM's* style.

Aside from all that, the articles themselves are something not usually seen in America any longer: long, well thought out, and planned; thoroughly researched with much background information; and factually presented. Where appropriate, all contain citations and references for follow-up research. Some of the material clearly pertains to Great Britain and will prove of less-than-passing interest. However, every issue contains both regular features and lengthy articles on alternative health that will prove of practical benefit. A few topics from recent issues include:

I Electromagnetism and cancer
I U.S. medical establishment
I Healing for professional health care practitioners.

Port Townsend Health Letter
Townsend Letter Group
911 Tyler Street
Port Townsend, WA 98368
206-385-4555

I Background

The *Port Townsend Health Letter*, a bimonthly ($6.50), four-page, informal letter, discusses in some detail nonallopathic, alternative therapies.

I What's Offered

Although written primarily for doctors, its straightforward style and jargon-free writing make it ideal for lay individuals interested in noninvasive therapies. Its motto; "Wellness Through Nutrition and Preventive Medicine," says it all.

Its short articles cover a wide arena of health, but primarily are concerned with alternative treatments for chronic degenerative diseases and common maladies. Although scholarly—all pieces are written by professional practitioners for other professionals—none of the material suffers from medical terminology-itis. And, even though literally speaking of life and death matters, humor and wit are not shunned but instead encouraged. A few of the topics that lay individuals might find of interest covered in recent issues are:

I Chelation therapy—studies for reversing heart and artery damage
I Chemotherapy—how it may cause cancer growth
I Nutritional profiles—individual needs
I Alternative cancer treatment study
I Weight management—using diet, nutrition, and exercise
I Stress evaluation—using psychological techniques
I Medical patients' rights—freedom of choice.

Solstice
310 East Main Street
Suite 105
Charlottesville, VA 22901
804-979-4427
804-979-1602 (fax)

I Background

Solstice, a monthly ($36), four-color magazine, offers practical information on natural foods, self-health, leading a macrobiotic lifestyle, and environmental concerns.

I What's Offered

Articles span the range of alternative health, nonorthodox treatments, cooking for health, environmental issues, and book reviews. All are served up informally but informatively. Regular monthly columns feature health through a natural lifestyle, natural foods news, updates on health and the environment, gardening organically, and cooking. Recent issues have had major articles on:

I Organic food certification
I Vitamin B_{12} for vegetarians
I Natural immunity through diet
I State dietician's licensing laws
I Cooking with soy for health
I Manmade viruses
I Organic baby food preparation
I Water filter comparisons
I Disposable versus washable diapers.

Each issue also has a directory of educational organizations, health and lifestyle network groups, and teaching centers as well as a reader service card.

Townsend Letter for Doctors
Townsend Letter Group
911 Tyler Street
Port Townsend, WA 98368
206-385-6021

I Background

The *Townsend Letter for Doctors*, published 10 times a year ($38), 100-page plus journal written by and for health care providers, is by far the most literate and scientific source for information about alternative healing and complementary medicine published in the United States.

I What's Offered

If you restrict yourself to a single source of information about alternative medicine, you could do worse than making it the

Townsend Letter. Both articles and critical letters come from around the world and are written by doctors: medical physicians, naturopaths, chiropractors, herbalists. There are no punches pulled. One month's article-length letters may be in response to a previous month's articles that some praise and others disagree with. The *Townsend Letter* is scholarly, technical, and filled with medical terms; nonetheless, you'll find almost everything in it fascinating and worth saving for years. All articles (and many letters) have references, some of which are organizations you can contact for more information and to locate a physician specializing in the therapy discussed. A tiny sample of the topics from recent issues are:

I Zinc and the prostate
I Scientific evaluation of prayer
I Germanium for the immune system
I Atherosclerosis and cow's milk
I Selenium toxicity
I Progesterone and premenstrual syndrome (PMS)
I Vegetable protein and diabetes
I Gut ecosystem dynamics.

Further Resources
Alternatives For The Health Conscious Individual
Choice
Healing Currents
Health and Healing
Hippocrates Health Institute
International Forum on New Science
Spectrum

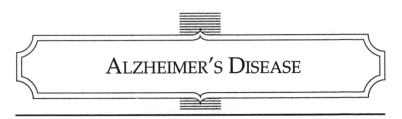

ALZHEIMER'S DISEASE

Alzheimer's Association
70 East Lake Street
Chicago, IL 60601-5997
800-621-0379
312-853-3060

■ Background

Alzheimer's is a degenerative disease attacking the brain. Its symptoms include severe memory loss, impaired thinking, and bizarre behavior. Four million American adults suffer from it; 10,000 of them die because of it every year.

No one knows what causes Alzheimer's. There isn't even a reliable clinical test for it. No cure exists although some alternative therapies show a decline in its severity.

The Alzheimer's Association:

- Organizes local support groups
- Supports research into causes and treatments
- Acts as an advocate for public policy and legislation.

■ What's Offered

The Association will direct you to one of its more than 200 chapters and 1600 local support groups nearest you. Its quarterly, *Alzheimer's Association Newsletter*, will keep you up-to-date on current research into causes, clinical studies of possible cures, and pending legislature affecting Alzheimer's.

Local support groups are most familiar with the care and treatment of Alzheimer's in their area. The one nearest you will help you with referrals to a practitioner.

American Health Assistance Foundation
15825 Shady Grove Road
Suite 140
Rockville, MD 20850
800-227-7998
301-258-9454 (fax)

▎Background

Retirement and growing older, once looked upon as the golden years, is now called the time of Alzheimer's disease. A quarter of a million Americans come down with this progressive, irreversible brain disorder each year; 100,000 of them will die from it. It is estimated that as many as 14 million Americans will get Alzheimer's within the next 50 years. Although its cause is unknown, current scientific research indicates that it may involve both a genetic predisposition along with several nongenetic or environment-related factors. A cure isn't even on the horizon.

The American Health Assistance Foundation (AHAF) supports research in the areas of Alzheimer's disease, glaucoma, and coronary heart disease.

▎What's Offered

The AHAF publishes a number of publications for the general public on Alzheimer's. They are all free, including the quarterly *Alzheimer's Research Review*. It is written for the average nonprofessional in nontechnical language, features readers' queries (and answers), and will provide you with information on the latest research finding and treatments.

The AHAF's toll-free number will provide you with information on the disease, identify alternative sources for help and support, answer any of your questions, and provide emotional support.

By the way, don't forget to ask for their information and free newsletters on glaucoma and heart disease as well.

Further Resources
   see all resources under CHELATION THERAPY

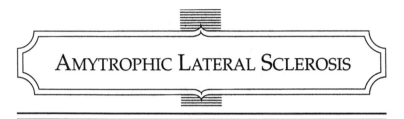

AMYTROPHIC LATERAL SCLEROSIS

Amytrophic Lateral Sclerosis Association
21021 Ventura Boulevard
Suite 321
Woodland Hills, CA 91364
800-782-4747 (hotline)
818-340-7500
818-340-2060 (fax)

Contact: Lynn M. Klein, Vice President, Patient Services

▌ Background

Amytrophic lateral sclerosis (ALS), more commonly known as Lou Gehrig's disease, is a neurological disorder characterized by progressive degeneration of the spinal cord and brain motor cells. Muscles are weakened, especially in the arms and legs. Speaking, swallowing, and breathing become difficult.

The ALS Association was formed to help patients and their families through:

- Education
- On-going research
- Support
- Information.

▌ What's Offered

The ALS Association has five self-help manuals on ALS for patients. They cover two main areas: finding additional help and coping with ALS and the difficulties involved with muscles, breathing, communicating, and swallowing.

A 12-page, tabloid-size newsletter, *Link*, is published quarerly. In it you will find articles gleaned from medical journals, upcoming events, news of local chapters, readers' queries, book and health care equipment reviews, and information on new research findings.

The Association has an unusual and extensive series of referral services with a large network of local chapters and support groups. These services include:

- Medical—physician, at-home services, hospital care
- Information—questions answered, further contacts
- Psychological support—volunteer counseling
- Resources—equipment for the handicapped.

The ALS Association has several regional clinical treatment centers, makes available several books to members, and keeps members informed of upcoming pharmaceutical and alternative treatment research in which they can take part.

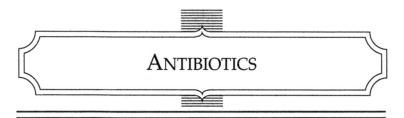

ANTIBIOTICS

Alliance for the Prudent Use of Antibiotics
P.O. Box 1372
Boston, MA 02117-1372
617-956-6765

Contact: Claire Sherman

▌ Background

Antibiotics are lifesavers. Since their introduction in the 1940s they have saved the lives of tens of millions of people. Antibiotics work by controlling and helping to prevent the spread of infectious bacterial diseases.

But today people are succumbing to diseases that were once treatable. New strains of bacteria are resistant to antibiotics that were once effective against them. It is no longer in dispute that these virulent strains are the direct result of antibiotic overuse and misuse.

Overuse of antibiotics from commonly available over-the-counter preparations, it is argued by many scientists and researchers, has made nearly all Americans less resistant to many of the diseases that have sprung up in the last few decades such as chronic fatigue syndrome and environmental illnesses.

The Alliance for the Prudent Use of Antibiotics (APUA) was formed to improve the understanding in both the health care community and among laypersons on antibiotic use and resistance.

▌ What's Offered

Although primarily a professional organization, membership ($35) in APUA is open to everyone and includes a subscription to the quarterly, eight-page *APUA Newsletter*. Nearly all the articles detail and document the adverse effects of antibiotic overuse and its resulting disease resistance.

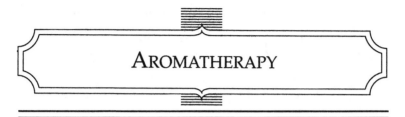

AROMATHERAPY

American Aromatherapy Association
P.O. Box 3679
South Pasedena, CA 91031
818-457-1742
818-300-8099 (fax)

▮ Background

Aromatherapy is one of the oldest medicinal uses of botanicals. Over 5000 years ago, ancient Egyptians used the scents of eucalyptus, lavender, and clove to treat skin disorders.

Aromatherapy is presently undergoing a renaissance in America. The publicity given to it by cosmetics researchers has made it common knowledge that the scent of spiced apples can lower blood pressure as much as a drug can.

Aromatherapy involves the use of aromatics extracted from stems, leaves, roots, flowers, and fruit. They heal both physical and psychological conditions when applied to the skin or inhaled through the nose.

The American Aromatherapy Association (AAA) is a professional organization of aromatherapists. As with most professional organizations, it helps to establish standards and to provide certification and training to its members.

▮ What's Offered

Although a professional organization, membership ($50) in AAA is open to the interested layperson.

AAA publishes a quarterly ($30), *Common Scents*. Journal articles discuss both technical aspects of aromatherapy and business matters relating to the profession. Recent articles on aromatherapy have discussed:

- Herbs and essential oils
- Lavender in skin care
- Ecology-oriented perfumes
- B'rth Respeth incense
- Helichrysum
- Analytic methods for essential oils.

The Association also maintains a directory of its members and will help you to locate a professional aromatherapist in your area.

International Journal of Aromatherapy
Essential Imports
401 Neptune Avenue
Suite B
Encinitas, CA 92024
619-944-8481

■ Background

Not suprisingly, aromatherapy is more highly regarded in Europe than in this country. So respected is it, that many licensed physicians and clinicians practice it.

The only scientifically based, medically based journal on the subject is the quarterly ($50) *International Journal of Aromatherapy*, published by the prestigious Tisserand Institute of Great Britain.

■ What's Offered

With an advisory board covering chemistry, biochemistry, pharmacology, botany, medical herbalism, general medicine, neurology, naturopathy, psychotherapy, psychology, and physiology, this prestigious journal bespeaks of scientific coverage of the subject. All the articles are technical—presumably to be read by professionals. Each subject is covered in depth: background, clinical and case studies, formulations, expected results. Most have references and citations culled from scientific literature. In short, this journal is for the devoted not the devoté. Recent topics of an alternative health bent include:

- Varicose veins
- Touch and pain
- Antimicrobial oils
- Chronic psoriasis
- Tea tree oil—acne
- Sense of smell and diagnosis.

National Association for Holistic Aromatherapy
P.O. Box 17622
Boulder, CO 80308-7622
303-258-3791

Background

Of the five senses—sight, touch, hearing, taste, and smell—smell is the one most neglected. Yet without its smell, a food loses its taste. Without a sense of smell, appetite often wanes. A single smell can often evoke vivid memories of childhood in even the oldest of people.

Botanical medicine, certainly the oldest form of therapy, is now joined by its country cousin, aromatherapy. We now know that aromatic substances, extracted from the flowers, stems, leaves, roots, or fruit of plants, can often heal; many are antiseptic and antifungal. More than 60 exhibit antibacterial properties.

When applied and then absorbed into the skin, these essential oils, as they are called, aid in healing muscular aches, arthritis symptoms, digestion, circulatory problems, and menstrual side effects. When inhaled through the nose, many of these oils trigger a reaction in the brain and can help people achieve numerous psychological effects. Stress becomes calmness, tension relaxation, and sorrow a feeling of joy.

The National Association for Holistic Aromatherapy (NAHA) is an organization of professional aromatherapists trained by the prestigious London School of Aromatherapy. All are certified by and members of the International Federation of Aromatherapists.

▌ What's Offered

A nonprofessional membership ($35) to NAHA entitles you to receive the Association's 12-page, quarterly newsletter, *Scentsitivity*. Its articles, though written for the profession, can be readily understood by the lay individual. Recent topics include such areas as:

- ▮ Essential oils
- ▮ Immunity
- ▮ Endometriosis
- ▮ Pregnancy.

The Association also maintains a referral list and will help you locate a professional aromatherapist in your area.

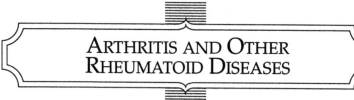

ARTHRITIS AND OTHER RHEUMATOID DISEASES

Rheumatoid Disease Foundation
5106 Old Harding Road
Franklin, TN 37064
615-646-1030

Contact: Perry A. Chapdelaine, Sr.

▌ Background

Arthritis, or joint inflammation, affects more than 36 million, or one in seven Americans. A new case is reported every 33 seconds. The two most common forms of arthritis are rheumatoid arthritis and osteoarthritis.

Conventional medicine claims that they are incurable: You must learn to live with the condition and take pain killers to alleviate its symptoms. Many alternative treatments say that not only can the pain be relieved, but that a cure is possible.

The Rheumatoid Disease Foundation (RDF) believes that it has found a successful series of alternative treatments; a cure or remission rate of 80% or better is claimed. Among the treatments are:

- Intraneural injections
- Hydrogen peroxide therapy
- Germanium
- Lactobacillus acidophilus—yogurt.

▌ What's Offered

In addition to promoting education on alternative treatments to professionals and laypersons and to conducting research at university centers, the RDF sells several publications outlining their treatment (many of the steps toward a cure can be done on your own) along with a physician and scientist advisory list (doctors who use the treatments in their practice).

––––––––

Further Resources
   see all resources under ENVIRONMENTAL ILLNESS
   see all resources under FOOD ALLERGIES
   American Apitherapy Society, Inc.

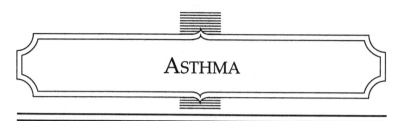

ASTHMA

National Asthma Education Program
4733 Bethesda Avenue
Suite 530
Bethesda, MD 20814

▌ Background

Asthma afflicts more than 10 million Americans. Yet, neither cause nor cure is known. Most mild sufferers use commonly prescribed antiasthma drugs known as beta 2-antagonists, while those with severe attacks generally rely on anti-inflammatory drugs. While these drugs, singly or in combination, relieve the symptoms of asthma, they often mask underlying causes of asthmatic attacks.

The National Asthma Education Program (NAEP) disseminates information on the risks of common asthma drugs and the benefits of simple, self-help steps that asthmatics can take.

▌ What's Offered

The major source of information from the NAEP is their report, *Guidelines for the Diagnosis and Management of Asthma*, available free. In it you will find information on the benefits and risks of common pharmaceuticals and general tips that can help lessen the severity of asthmatic attacks such as indoor environmental dangers. Dust mites, pet dander and saliva, insect parts, and mold are all known to trigger severe attacks.

National Foundation for Asthma, Inc.
5301 East Grant Road
Tucson, AZ 85712
602-323-6046

■ Background

Many people have tightness and a heavy feeling in their chest and shortness of breath. They also wheeze and cough. A good many of them may suffer from asthma without knowing it.

The myths surrounding who gets asthma, what asthma is, what asthmatics may or may not physically do, and what self-help steps they can take are rampant. For instance, asthma is not psychosomatic, contagious, or a children's disease. Neither do all asthmatics eventually get emphysema. In fact, of all the old wives' tales about asthma only one is true: chicken soup helps. Medical studies have shown that the hot chicken soup thins nasal and chest congestion, which makes it easier to clear the excess mucus. You see, your mother really was right about chicken soup when she said "it's what's good for you!"

The National Foundation for Asthma, Inc., affiliated with the Tucson Medical Center Chest Clinic, also makes available information about asthma to the general public.

■ What's Offered

Supported solely by contributions, two of their little, pocketbook-sized booklets, *Asthma: Fact and Fiction* and *Dust n' Stuff*, will provide anyone concerned about asthma with useful, self-help facts. Several other booklets discuss allergens specific to southern Arizona.

Asthma: Fact and Fiction will explain how your lungs work, and will tell you of the symptoms that may indicate asthma, the types and possible contributing causes of asthma, and what you and your doctor can do to alleviate some of the more debilitating symptoms. *Dust n' Stuff* will help you to allergy-proof your home with dozens of easy-to-do things that will eliminate many of the common irritants and environmental factors that trigger an attack and make it more devastating. For example, a 1991 University of Kentucky study showed that about 60% of asthmatics were so allergic to the garden-variety of cockroach that they suffered severe asthmatic attacks.

Further Resources
  see all resources under RESPIRATORY ILLNESSES

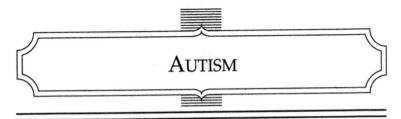

AUTISM

Autism Research Institute
4182 Adams Avenue
San Diego, CA 92116
619-281-7165

Contact: Bernard Rimland, Director

▌ Background

Autism is a severe behavioral disorder striking children soon after birth. It is characterized by an inability to relate to or communicate with other people. Some autistics are mute, others speak in a strange ritualistic manner.

The Autism Research Institute (ARI) conducts independent research in the use of high dosages of vitamin B6 and magnesium as a treatment for many of the symptoms. This orthomolecular approach stresses the autistic's profound need or poor utilization of these nutrients. ARI's additional research is conducted in the areas of:

- Psychology
- Neurology
- Genetics
- Biochemistry
- Nutrition
- Vitamins.

■ What's Offered

ARI publishes a quarterly journal, *Autism Research Review International*, that reviews its own and others' research results, clinical case studies, and new treatments for autism and other autistic-related disorders.

For a nominal $1, ARI will send you literature on the causes and treatment of autism, including its own research findings. This includes several treatments of choice:

■ Orthomolecular—megavitamin therapy
■ Junk food–free diets
■ Avoidance of psychotherapy and drugs.

ARI has an exhaustive publication list on a variety of alternative therapies for autism and refers patients and their families to alternative health care professionals and clinics offering holistic treatments for both autism and other childhood nerve disorders.

Autism Services Center
Prichard Building
605 9th Street
P.O. Box 507
Huntington, WV 25710-0507
304-525-8014
304-525-8026 (fax)

■ Background

While everyone knows that autism affects children, its symptoms last for as long as autistics live—a lifetime of extreme aloneness and unresponsiveness to other people based on an inability to understand and to use language.

The Autism Services Center (ASC) assists families of autistic children and acts as an advocate with technical assistance in designing appropriate therapy.

▌ What's Offered

The ASC also publishes a six-page quarterly, *Behind the Lines*. It is filled with stories of autistics who have benefited from different therapies as well as news of the Center's treatment facilities.

Hardly advocating strictly alternative therapies, the ASC nevertheless provides information on a wide range of available training and therapeutic options, including many safe, non-pharmaceutical ones.

Autism Society of America
8601 Georgia Avenue
Suite 503
Silver Springs, MD 20910
301-565-0433
301-565-0834 (fax)

▌ Background

Autism—severe, incapacitating, developmental disability that starts at birth—strikes five out of every 10,000 children.

The Autism Society of America (ASA) provides information about autism and its various treatment modalities to the parents of autistic children.

▌ What's Offered

Affiliated with 160 local support groups, the ASA believes that special education, supportive counseling, and a controlled diet provide the best treatment at present and will provide answers to difficult problems relating to autism or autistic-like conditions.

A $20 annual membership will entitle you to their 20-page, quarterly newsletter, *The Advocate*. Much of the information is supportive in nature, but news of new treatments and research findings are also discussed. Many of the articles are written by local chapter members, and the magazine has no fixed format. Regular features include readers' letters and a resource information exchange.

ASA also makes available a wide range of books on autism and dealing with autistic children.

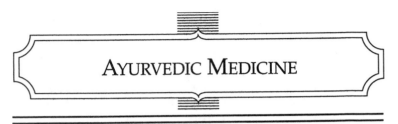

AYURVEDIC MEDICINE

Maharishi Ayur-Veda Association of America
P.O. Box 282
Fairfield, IA 52556
515-472-8477

Contact: Evelyn Shatkin

▌Background

India is one of the oldest civilizations still in existence. As such, its medical and health care traditions have survived the test of time. Unquestionably, these healing arts have proved beneficial to many millions more than all modern medicine has.

Ayurvedic medicine is one of India's most comprehensive systems of natural medicine and is recognized as effective by the United Nation's World Health Organization. Recently this treatment modality has been revived in the United States and has been made an adjunct of transcendental meditation. The resulting system is more clinical in its approach to health and disease than the original Indian version.

The Maharishi Ayur-Veda Association of America, aside from its regional clinics, sponsors medical conferences on Ayurvedic medicine for medical professionals, and its members contribute to peer-reviewed medical and scientific journals.

▌What's Offered

In general terms, the ayurvedic approach consists of 20 approaches to such Western ailments as stress, poor diet, lack of exercise, and poor nutrition. The three major goals of this blend, called Maharishi Ayur-Veda, are:

∎ To prevent and treat disease
∎ To preserve health
∎ To promote longevity.

Through its nine regional centers and several dozen local health centers, the Association's treatment method offers personal initial evaluations followed by rejuvenation therapy. Treatments, many of which can be done at home, include diet, exercise, daily and seasonal health routines, herbal supplements, neuromuscular and neurorespiratory programs, and stress management.

Additionally, educational material on ayurvedic as well as Indian herbal supplements that help with specific body imbalances and focus on strengthening the entire physiology, may also be ordered.

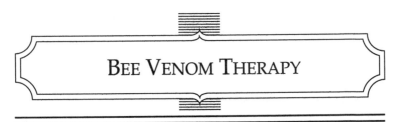

BEE VENOM THERAPY

American Apitherapy Society, Inc.
34 Heron Road
Middletown, NJ 07748
201-671-5877

Contact: Dr. Christopher M. Kim, President

▌ Background

Apitherapy is the therapeutic use of honey bee venom and honey bee products. Although neither recognized nor much used in America, bee venom is both used and respected as a therapy in Western Europe. (German physicians often prescribe a prepared dose of refrigerated bee venom therapy to permanently reduce arthritic swelling and pain.) It is not uncommon treatment in Russia and the Ukraine for many inflammatory ailments.

The American Apitherapy Society, Inc., is an organization of professionals and lay individuals promoting the use of and conducting research into the therapeutic uses of bees and their venom.

▌ What's Offered

The Society provides technical and clinical information, conducts and supports original research on bee venom therapy, and holds an annual convention. It publishes a quarterly newsletter on the curative properties and therapeutic uses of honey bee venom in human medicine, which is available by subscription.

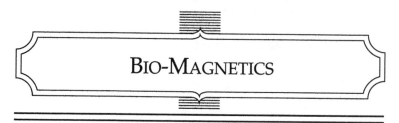

Bio-Magnetics

Albert Roy Davis Research Laboratory
P.O. Box 655
Green Cove Springs, FL 32043
904-264-8564

■ Background

Energy and matter make up and pervade the universe. This means that not only are we material beings but beings of energy—magnetic and electromagnetic energy. In fact, many of the basic molecules that make up life are tiny magnets; each has a north pole and a south pole and exhibit all the properties of other magnets.

Coming down to us from ancient history are tales of electrical and magnetic healing. But only recently—in the last 50 years—has scientific investigation been applied to this phenomenon.

The Albert Roy Davis Research Laboratory disseminates information on its own unique research findings in the field of biomagnetics and magnetic healing.

■ What's Offered

Many books written by the researchers and specially prepared reports are available on subjects such as the effect of magnetism on life, using magnets to diagnose illnesses, and healing a variety of disorders with magnets.

Several types of specially prepared magnets and magnetic products are also available.

Bio-Electro-Magnetics Institute
2490 West Moana Lane
Reno, NV 89509-3936
702-827-9099

Contact: Dr. John T. Zimmerman, President

▌ Background

Although pharmaceuticals and surgical intervention constitute the major treatments of most ailments today, their days may be numbered. As physics and biochemistry delve below the molecular level, they find we are beings of magnetism and electricity. In other words, humans are biomagnetic as well as biological.

The field of biomagnetism is so new in science that even basic definitions are in dispute. Nevertheless, there are two components to it: the study of the electrical and magnetic fields within and surrounding living organisms and investigation of how external electric and magnetic fields (especially manmade ones) affect life.

The Bio-Electro-Magnetics Institute (BEMI) conducts basic and applied research into biomagnetism.

▌ What's Offered

Besides its research, BEMI publishes *BEMI Currents*, a quarterly ($40), 24-page newsletter. Articles are written by recognized experts and scientists in the field and are usually accompanied by references for further research. Article topics run the gamut in the field: the dangers of electromagnetic fields from power lines and video display terminals, magnetic healing, full-spectrum lighting, and structured water. A sample of recent article topics includes:

- ▌ Bioenergetic medicine
- ▌ Patient reports of pulsed magnetic field therapy
- ▌ Electromagnetism and polarity therapy
- ▌ Chi and energy medicine

■ Bioelectromagnetic communication
■ Health benefits of natural sunlight and full-spectrum lighting
■ Critical review of magnetotherapy.

BEMI also conducts tests at locations across the country to investigate whether there are dangerous electromagnetic fields present and offers guidance in reducing their dangers or eliminating them.

Enviro -Tech Products
17171 S.E. 29th Street
Choctaw, OK 73020
405-390-3499

■ Background

Not only have research and clinical data shown that magnetics can have a profound effect upon health and disease, but evidence suggests that the magnetic forces themselves are more complex than previously thought. For example, some scientists believe that there is no difference between the two magnetic poles; the north and south poles are identical and one is designated positive and the other negative merely for the sake of convenience.

But both the initial research of Albert Roy Davis and Walter C. Rawls, Jr., and the subsequent work of Dr. William Philpott suggest otherwise. They have discovered that the magnetic north pole has a beneficial effect upon health and the south pole a harmful effect. The implication of this is profound when one thinks of the billions of dollars spent on fancy diagnostic hardware and pharmaceuticals, not to mention the pain and suffering that could be relieved.

Enviro-Tech's products are the result of Dr. Philpott's initial research on magnetic therapy. The design of the products and their marketing are based on his advice.

▌ What's Offered

Several of Philpott's books on magnetic therapy, diabetes, and allergies, as well as an extensive collection of specially developed magnetic products are available. Additionally, Philpott has prepared several reports on the use of magnets in diagnosing and healing a wide variety of common ailments.

Resonance
P.O. Box 64
Sumterville, FL 33585
904-793-8748

Contact: Judy Wall

▌ Background

Bioelectromagnetics is the science of the interaction between electrical and magnetic fields and living organisms. The use of both permanent and electric magnets to relieve pain, stimulate the immune system, and even cure chronic conditions is widely accepted as valid in many countries and practiced extensively in Japan.

Resonance is the quarterly publication of a special interest group of MENSA (an organization of persons who have scored 98% or above on any standard IQ test).

▌ What's Offered

A year's subscription to *Resonance* is $6. Its articles, reviews, and questions serve more as a way to communcicate between people who have an interest in the subject than as a means of finding practical applications for biomagnetics.

Further Resources
Foundation for Research of Natural Therapies

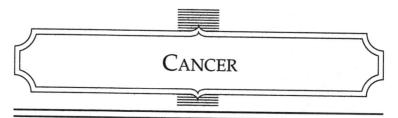

CANCER

American Institute for Cancer Research
Development Office
1759 R Street, NW
Washington, DC 20070-2012
800-843-8114
202-328-7744

∎ Background

Not all orthodox medicine ignores or downplays what the alternative health care community has said for decades: that there is a link between diet and cancer. Specifically, as it applies to us all, the link is that diet and nutrition can help prevent cancer.

The American Institute for Cancer Research (AICR) not only funds hundreds of research projects on nutrition and cancer but also provides information to both physicians and the general public.

∎ What's Offered

The AICR provides a variety of services for consumers:

∎ A toll-free nutrition hotline to answer personal questions about good nutrition and good health
∎ A series of consumer seminars in 24 cities on reducing cancer risk
∎ The *AICR Newsletter*: a quarterly, four-page newsletter with articles on research updates, health tips for consumers, recipes and meal planning, and nutrition ideas about eating and better health

- Four seasonal cookbooks featuring recipes from appetizers to desserts that follow cancer risk-reduction dietary guidelines
- Video on nutrition and cancer
- A series of free, colorful educational booklets on dietary guidelines to lower cancer risk.

The AICR also has a special Physician's Information Program that supplies doctors' offices with AICR educational booklets.

Arlin J. Brown Information Center, Inc.
P.O. Box 251
Fort Belvoir, VA 22060
703-451-8638

Contact: Arlin J. Brown

▌ Background

The Arlin J. Brown Information Center, Inc. is a clearinghouse for information on natural, nontoxic treatments for chronic and degenerative diseases, with special emphasis on cancer.

▌ What's Offered

A $25 membership will get you a subscription to their monthly, four-page newsletter, *Health Victory Bulletin*. Each issue, instead of discussing many subjects, focuses on a single topic. All the articles are clearly written, concise without leaving vital information out, and documented with clinical studies. Further sources of information on where to purchase the recommended nutrients and where to obtain more information are also given. Some recent topics are:

- Coenzyme Q_{10}

- Anticancer effects of barley leaves
- Ozone and AIDS
- Mucopolysaccharides and arthritis
- Koch treatment and glyoxylide
- Wheatgrass diet
- Cancer and arthritis.

A directory of clinics and health care practitioners (many are M.D.'s, some are O.D.'s and N.D.'s) who use nutritional and non-toxic treatments and diagnostic tests is also available. Many reprints of articles from a variety of international magazines and journals on a wide range of diseases and their cures through natural means are also available.

Cancer Control Society
2043 North Berendo Street
Los Angeles, CA 90027
213-663-7801

Contact: Lorraine Rosenthal

▎ Background

Many, if not most, alternative health care organizations are devoted to promoting the benefits of a particular treatment methodology.

The Cancer Control Society (CCS), a nonprofit information and education organization, takes an eclectic approach to alternative therapies: Whatever seems to work should be explored and available to whoever desires it.

■ What's Offered

The CCS provides many services. Membership ($25) includes a directory of alternative treatment clinics and a subscription to the bimonthly magazine, *Cancer Control Journal*. Each issue's articles discuss a variety of therapies for cancer and cancer prevention techniques and include profiles on many clinics utilizing them. The magazine is not limited exclusively to cancer; many articles can be found on arthritis, heart problems, cataracts, glaucoma, and multiple sclerosis. Recent topics have included:

- Health benefits of raw vegetables
- Enzyme–cancer connection
- Homeopathy and cancer
- Ozone therapy
- Electromagnetic treatments
- Nutritional control of cataracts
- Hyperthermia and cancer control
- Natural treatments for chronic fatigue syndrome.

Associated with the Society is an annual two- or three-day conference at which recognized experts discuss a variety of therapies and preventive techniques directed toward the general public. For those unable to attend, all conventions are available on audio tape.

The CCS also runs the Cancer Book House. This bookstore has an extensive collection of books, reprints, and videos from all over the world on nutrition, cancer, and many other nutrition-related disorders.

Additional services include a 24-hour hotline and a referral service to alternative health care practitioners and clinics.

Cancer Research Institute
133 East 58th Street
New York, NY 10022
800-99-CANCER
212-688-7515

▌Background

Cancer, one of the scariest sounding words to most people, refers to approximately 150 different diseases. Their commonality is an uncontrolled growth of cells and the ability to enter and damage normal tissues.

Some degree of immune response to cancer exists in us all. Our immune system works by defending the body against any foreign substance. If that were not so, the human race would die out in less than a week.

The Cancer Research Institute (CRI) funds research in increasing the body's immune response to cancer through the development of immune response modifiers, monoclonial antibodies, and vaccines. The advantage of using the body's own immune system could lead to a more natural approach than the conventionally accepted treatments of surgery, radiation, and chemotherapy.

▌What's Offered

Supported solely by contributions, the CRI, in addition to its research, publishes and distributes free of charge a quarterly, four-page newsletter of recent highlights of new developments in cancer, immunology, and AIDS called *Science Highlights*. In it you will find mostly conventional medical news, although some unorthodox treatments are also covered. What they all have in common is their ability to increase the body's own immune system in response to disease.

Foundation for Advancement in Cancer Therapy
P.O. Box 1242
Old Chelsea Station
New York, NY 10113
212-741-2790

Contact: Ruth Sackman

▌ Background

The war on cancer was officially declared in 1971. Many billions of dollars and lives later, Harvard University biostatistician John Bailar III stated in the prestigious *New England Journal of Medicine* of May 1986 that the war was lost.

The Foundation for Advancement in Cancer Therapy (FACT) is an educational organization, established to act as an information clearinghouse for cancer information, and a referral service.

▌ What's Offered

FACT does not advocate any therapies, orthodox or alternative. Instead, they seek a reevaluation of cancer as a systemic disease rather than a specific one. Believing in treating the entire person rather than just the disease, they fall (in spite of their own protestations to the contrary) on the holistic side of health care and include:

- Early noninvasive diagnosis
- Nutrition
- Detoxification
- Structural imbalance
- Mind–body connection
- Nontoxic programs including fever therapy, immunotherapy, cellular therapy, and botanicals.

Contributions of $10 (or more) include a subscription to *Cancer Forum*, FACT's newsletter that reports on new approaches to diagnosing and treating cancer.

FACT also holds several conferences on new discoveries in cancer: its treatment and prevention. Recent topics of a conference entitled "Host Resistance" included:

- Metabolic treatment modalities
- Natural healing
- Cellular therapy
- Oriental medicine
- Nutritional approaches.

A catalogue of books, reprint articles, and audio tapes will also be sent.

FACT goes out of its way to not make specific referrals or recommendations to health care practitioners. However, they will supply you with the resources and the data to help you to make your own decision.

Gerson Institute
P.O. Box 430
Bonita, CA 92002
619-267-1150

▌ Background

For many years the Gerson Institute has provided a successful, intensive, nutrition-based therapy for a variety of life-threatening, chronic conditions, especially cancer.

▮ What's Offered

In addition to treating patients, the Institute also offers many books, audio tapes, videos, and a quarterly ($15) newsletter, *The Healing Newsletter* and holds conventions and seminars. The topics covered in all this material is wide-ranging and clearly alternative. Recent topics have dealt with:

- Sunlight and health
- Lymphatic system—trapped blood proteins
- Thyroid therapy—heart disease
- Diet and cancer—prevention, cure
- Healing clays and herbs—absorbing toxins
- Disease prevention through food.

International Association of Cancer Victors and Friends, Inc.
7740 West Manchester
Suite 110
Playa del Rey, CA 90291
213-822-5032

▮ Background

Despite the billions of dollars spent on cancer research, despite the claims of conventional medical treatments, cancer rates are going up.

The International Association of Cancer Victors and Friends, Inc. was started by a cancer victor, not a cancer victim—a woman who conquered cancer by using nontoxic therapies instead of chemotherapy and drugs. Its goals are:

- To educate the public about unconventional, nontoxic therapies and known cancer-causing substances
- To help physicians get the right to prescribe these therapies

■ To act as an information center
■ To collect and disseminate new information about alternative cancer treatments.

■ What's Offered

Your $20 membership entitles you to receive a list of recovered patients to contact about their cancer and treatment, nontoxic therapy and diagnostic directory, and a list of treatment centers.

You will also receive the Association's quarterly newsletter, *Cancer Victors Journal*. The journal provides personal stories from recovered cancer patients, news of alternative therapies, promising laboratory tests, nutrition news, and news of conventional medical breakthroughs.

Linus Pauling Institute of Science and Medicine
440 Page Mill Road
Palo Alto, CA 94306-2025
415-327-4064
415-327-8564 (fax)

Contact: Richard Hicks, Executive Vice President

■ Background

The Linus Pauling Institute of Science and Medicine does extensive research on the use of vitamin C and other nutrients in the treatment and prevention of cancer and other degenerative diseases, AIDS, cholesterol and diet, and the molecular investigation of aging.

▌What's Offered

The Institute also publishes a quarterly newsletter and an extensive array of research reports and booklets on alternative treatments of diseases and preventive techniques. The newsletter provides health information on on-going medical research projects undertaken by the Institute. Recent issues discussed are:

- Tumor regression—diet and nutrient therapy
- Use of intravenous ascorbate in cancer
- AIDS and nutrition—megadose therapy
- Recent research on vitamin C
- Coenzyme Q_{10} and heart disease
- Dietary phytate (found in whole grains) in slowing tumor growth and lowering cholesterol.

Also available from the Institute are several of Pauling's books and lecture series, including:

- *Cancer and Vitamin C*
- *How to Live Longer and Feel Better*
- "Surgery: Your Choices, Your Alternatives"
- "Symposium, Volume I—Nutrition, Health and Peace."

Note: Please see the second listing for the Linus Pauling Institute under HEART DISEASE, HIGH BLOOD PRESSURE, and STROKE for important information.

Nutrition and Cancer
Lawrence Erlbaum Associates
365 Broadway
Hillsdale, NJ 07642
201-666-4110
201-666-2394 (fax)

▌ Background

Nutrition and Cancer, a biannual journal ($120), is too costly for all but the most avid reader of health information.

▌ What's Offered

The reports are technical and the language scholarly (although thankfully free from most jargon). The information, however, may be worth the effort if you have a serious interest in how nutrition can affect and prevent the onslaught of cancer.

If you take the time to read the articles, even to read the abstracts and conclusions, you will soon see the effect of diet and nutrients on both cancer risk and cancer treatment. For convincing evidence just look at this list of recent topics:

- Dietary fiber and breast cancer risk
- Diet and gastric cancer
- Colon cancer and fiber
- Selenium and cancer
- Milk consumption and cancer risk
- Dietary factors and lymphoma
- Alcohol intake and rectal cancer risks.

Visit your local medical school to get a look at *Cancer and Nutrition*. Not only are you likely to find this journal, but many of the others discussed in this book.

Patient Advocates for Advanced Cancer Treatments, Inc.
1143 Parmelee NW
Grand Rapids, MI 49504-1695
616-453-1477

Contact: Lloyd J. Ney

▌ Background

The Patient Advocates for Advanced Cancer Treatments, Inc., unlike other organizations devoted to studying cancer causes and treatments, is actually a national support group. It focuses on making unconventional treatments legal and available.

▌ What's Offered

A $25 membership includes a subscription to the newsletter, *Cancer Communication*, a monthly, 12-page magazine. A recent issue, aside from letters to the editor, news of local support groups, and legal matters relating to recent court rulings and legislature, had short articles on:

- Prostate cancer
- Timely medical news of various cancers
- Hypothermia treatment
- Radiology testing
- Blood tests
- The benefits of L-carnitine
- Flutamide therapy
- RU 486
- Cancer insurance.

People Against Cancer
P.O. Box 10
Otho, IA 50569-0010
515-972-4444
Contact: Frank D. Wiewel, President

▌ Background

People Against Cancer (PAC) is dedicated to protecting medical freedom of choice; specifically as it relates to cancer therapies. PAC does this by distributing a wide range of literature on alternative, nontoxic cancer therapies; preventive lifestyles; the political aspects of cancer; and home health care products.

▌ What's Offered

Yearly membership ($25) to PAC includes the bimonthly newsletter, *The Cancer Chronicles*. Recent issues have included articles on:

- Cancer and the poor
- Antineoplastons—an alternative treatment
- Selenium—deficiencies
- Interleukin-2 and kidney cancer
- Hydrazine sulfate—a complementary therapy
- Immune therapy.

  Additional services provided include:

- Regional seminars to help those with cancer to form self-help and support groups
- Speakers for local groups and conventions
- Counseling service
- An extensive list of educational materials, including books, articles, audio tapes, and videos.

  PAC also provides a counseling service for those seeking guidance in choosing alternative therapies.

RECNAC/Project
Bio-Communications Research Institute
3100 North Hillside Avenue
Wichita, KS 67219
316-682-3100
316-682-5054 (fax)

▌ Background

There are a host of effective alternative therapies for cancer. Many are complex biochemical formulations, some are eclectic, borrowing features from several treatments; others are simple but strict nutrititional approaches. Yet no rigorous scientific research on cellular nutrition, cancer, and biocommunications has been undertaken.

That is the stated purpose of the 10-year RECNAC (Research Encompassing Comprehensive Novel Approaches to Cancer) Project—to develop a treatment protocol for the treatment and prevention of cancer through nutrients.

▌ What's Offered

To help support its work, the Project publishes an eight page, monthly newsletter, *Health Hunter*. All its short articles are written by professionals and discuss practical applications of information on nutrients, relaxation techniques, lifestyle changes and other alternative approaches to disease prevention and treatment. Some recent topics have included:

- ▌ Vitamins—cancer prevention
- ▌ Secondhand tobacco smoke and cancer
- ▌ Trees and healing
- ▌ Fish oil—triglyceride reduction
- ▌ Antioxidants—nutritional defense against cancer
- ▌ Comfrey
- ▌ Weight control—breakthrough approaches

▮ Exercising in polluted areas.

Several books on alternative healing are also available.

Further Resources
see all references under OXIDATIVE THERAPIES
Exceptional Cancer Patients
Nutrition Education Association, Inc.

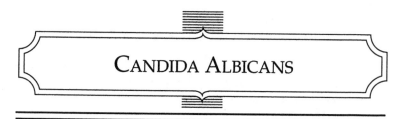

CANDIDA ALBICANS

Candida Research and Information Foundation
P.O. Box 2719
Castro Valley, CA 94546
415-582-2179

∎ Background

Candidiasis, until very recently, was not considered a disease. Presenting their symptoms to a physician, sufferers were met with disbelief and then told to see a psychiatrist, grow up, have an affair, or get a job, or they were laughed at.

The Candida Research and Information Foundation, a grassroots informal organization, provides information to help candidiasis sufferers.

∎ What's Offered

The Foundation's monthly newsletter follows no fixed format. Written in an informal style, you are as likely to find excerpts from a medical symposium or the findings of clinical studies as a product review. What is always present is pertinent and practical information:

- ∎ Recommended reading lists
- ∎ Support group informat on
- ∎ Case histories
- ∎ Research findings
- ∎ Product reviews
- ∎ Alternative therapies.

International Health Federation
P.O. Box 3494
Jackson, TN 38302
901-427-8100

Contact: Sally Karlgaard-Harvey, R.N.

▌Background

Candida albicans is a series of yeast-related infectious disorders that primarily affect women.
The International Health Federation (IHF) provides information on candidiasis to the general public.

▌What's Offered

Information from the IHF is available in several formats. If you send a self-addressed, stamped envelope plus $1 you will receive general literature on the various forms of candidiasis and some of its symptoms. A bound compendium of reprints, excerpts, letters to the editor, and reports from the scientific literature such as the *Journal of the American Medical Association* and *Hospital Practice* is available for $50. The articles are written by such highly regarded experts on yeast-related illnesses as C. Orian Truss, M.D.; Steven S. Witkin, Ph.D.; Kasuo Iwata, M.D.; E. W. Rosenberg, M.D.; Sidney M. Baker, M.D.; and Martin W. Zwerling, M.D. An unbound abbreviated version of the compendium is avaiable for $15.

The Federation operates a hotline from 11 A.M. to 12 P.M. CST. When you telephone, your questions on yeast-related infections will be answered by a trained and knowledgeable professional.

Direct referrals are not given, However, if you send a self-addressed, stamped envelope plus $5 to the IHF c/o Susan Yarborough, you will be sent the names of physicians in your area who have experience treating yeast-related disorders.

Further Resources
Allergy Alert

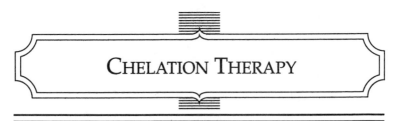

CHELATION THERAPY

American Board of Chelation Therapy
70 West Huron Street
Chicago, IL 60610
312-787-ABCT

▌ Background

The American Board of Chelation Therapy (ABCT) is a professional organization of physicians and scientists who have successfully undertaken advanced training in chelation therapy. Chelation therapy consists of intravenous injections of a prescription medicine known as EDTA.

Although currently FDA approved for removing heavy metals such as lead, mercury, and cadmium from the body, EDTA is currently being tested under the auspices of the FDA for treatment of atherosclerosis, or hardening of the arteries.

▌ What's Offered

ABCT members, called Diplomates, are also members of the American College of Advanced Medicine. Most medical and health-related questions are better answered by the American College of Advancement in Medicine. But if you are considering chelation therapy, you may wish that your physician also be a member of ABCT.

Additionally, if you have any medical questions relating to chelation therapy that remain unanswered from ACAM, the ABCT is the place to get the answers.

American College of Advancement in Medicine
23121 Verdugo Drive
Suite 204
Laguna Hills, CA 92653
800-LEAD-OUT
714-583-7666

▌ Background

Chelation therapy consists of intravenous injections of a prescription medicine called EDTA. EDTA is currently approved for removing heavy metals such as lead, mercury, and cadmium from the body.

The American College of Advancement in Medicine (ACAM) is a professional organization of physicians and scientists who believe and practice alternative medicine, including nutritional counseling, supplementary nutrients, and chelation therapy.

ACAM believes and offers strong clinical evidence that EDTA can also reverse the symptoms of atherosclerosis, or hardening of the arteries.

▌ What's Offered

An inquiry will bring you a pamphlet on chelation therapy, explaining:

- What chelating is
- EDTA—what it is
- How chelation therapy affects overall health
- Safety and side effects of chelation therapy
- Benefits of chelation therapy
- Insurance coverage of treatment.

Also included is a list of several dozen technical and general books on chelation therapy that you may order.

The College maintains a membership directory. If asked, they will include a list of several physicians in your area who have received extensive training in chelation therapy and have been board-certified by the American Board of Chelation Therapy.

ACAM's official publication is the *Journal of Advancement in Medicine*, published by Human Sciences Press, Inc., in New York City. It is meant only for members and concentrates primarily on technical discussions and clinical practices of chelation therapy.

ACAM also holds several conferences a year on other chronic conditions and a variety of atherosclerosis therapies such as cellular treatment, prostaglandins, mercury detoxification, parasites, detoxification, and magnesium therapy.

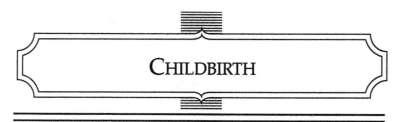

CHILDBIRTH

American Academy of Husband-Coached Childbirth
P.O. Box 5224
Sherman Oaks, CA 91413-5224
800-423-2397

Contact: Dr. Robert A. Bradley

▌ Background

Natural childbirth is much in demand by parents-to-be. Birthing, as it is called, is looked upon as an experience to be shared between husband and wife. However, physicians and midwives find that those parents know little of natural childbirth and require classroom training.

The Bradley Method of coached childbirth, taught by the American Academy of Husband-Coached Childbirth (AAHCC), stresses the following:

- Natural childbirth
- Active participation of the husband as a coach
- Nutrition
- Avoidance of drugs
- Breastfeeding
- Relaxation and natural breathing
- Parental responsibility.

▌ What's Offered

If you write or telephone, the AAHCC will send you a brochure containing:

- Contents of the 12-lesson course taught to husbands and wives around the country
- A national directory of all certified and trained instructors to help you find one in your area
- Information on books and videos you may buy that will tell you more about many aspects of natural childbirth.

American College of Nurse-Midwives
1522 K Street, NW
Washington, DC 20005
202-289-0171
202-289-4395 (fax)

Contact: Diane Say

▌ Background

A certified nurse-midwife is trained in both nursing and midwifery and helps the mother:

- Before and after pregnancy—advice about reproductive health, conception, personal care; provides gynecological services such as pelvic and breast exams and pap smears
- During pregnancy—monitoring her health and that of her baby and providing educational advice on nutrition, exercise, childbirth methods, and infant health
- During labor—evaluating its progress and offering emotional and physical support while facilitating the natural labor process

- At birth—assisting delivery and examining the newborn baby
- After delivery—providing follow-up care and advice on self-care, breast or bottle feeding, and infant care.

The American College of Nurse-Midwives (ACNM) is a professional organization and certifying agency of nurse-midwives.

What's Offered:

The ACNM offers books and pamphlets on nurse-midwife general information, its clinical practice, legal information, and the education required to be a professional nurse-midwife.

They will also provide you with a referral to a certified nurse-midwife in your area or answer any questions you might have concerning nurse-midwifery.

ASPO/Lamaze
1840 Wilson Boulevard
Suite 204
Arlington, VA 22201
800-368-4404
703-524-7802

Background

ASPO, standing for the American Society for Psychoprophylaxis in Obstetrics, is a professional organization of childbirth educators that focuses on:

- Education—for families and health care professionals
- Advocacy—alternative childbirth, care, and maternal–child health

■ Reform—legislating alternative childbirth for those wanting it.

■ What's Offered

ASPO's 30 chapters throughout the United States make it easy for interested families to take childbirth preparation classes from trained instructors where they will learn:

■ Lamaze relaxation techniques
■ Anatomy and physiology of pregnancy, labor, and delivery
■ Nutrition during pregnancy
■ Comfort during labor
■ Drug, alcohol, and tobacco avoidance
■ Risks and benefits of childbirth medications
■ Labor variations, complications, and cesareans
■ Evaluating birth choices
■ Breastfeeding and bottle feeding
■ Infant care and bonding
■ Postpartum.

ASPO also maintains and makes available to anyone interested a national referral service to over 9000 childbirth educators and companions.

Association for Childbirth At Home, International
P.O. Box 430
Glendale, CA 91209
213-667-0839

■ Background

Very few newborns arrive in this world in hospitals. Those who are born in the homes of their parents have a higher survival rate and fewer health problems than those born in hospitals or maternity centers.

The Association for Childbirth At Home, International (ACH) disseminates information to prospective parents and professionals interested in home childbirth.

▌ What's Offered

Besides an extensive library of reference material on homebirth and individual consultation, ACH's six-session training falls into the following broad categories:

- ▌ Advantages of homebirth
- ▌ Normal birth process
- ▌ Psychological issues
- ▌ Medical considerations
- ▌ Preparations for birth
- ▌ Newborn.

A referral service to physicians, nurses, and midwives who assist in homebirth is also available.

Childbirth Without Pain Education Association
20134 Snowden
Detroit, MI 48235
313-341-3816

▌ Background

To many women, the pain of chilbirth may be the worst pain they have ever felt. Yet it is possible to have a painless birth experience, for the father to share in that experience, and for the baby to get a safe delivery.

The method is called the psychoprophylactic (or Lamaze) method and involves four people: the Lamaze teacher, the expectant parents, and their physician or midwife.

The Childbirth Without Pain Education Association (CWPEA) maintains its own educational center to instruct expectant parents in the Lamaze method, trains other teachers, and engages in research on painless childbirth.

▌ What's Offered

The six classes offered by CWPEA first decondition the mother to expect pain and then teach a new type of labor contraction that will eliminate the pain.

Lamaze teachers are trained by the CWPEA and a referral to a teacher in your area may be obtained by telephoning or writng.

Consumers Advocating the Legalization of Midwifery
P.O. Box 7902
Citrus Heights, CA 95621-7902
916-791-7831

Contact: Anita Butler, President

▌ Background

While other CHILDBIRTH resources in this book speak of midwifery as a birthing option, this one addresses something even more fundamental: your right to have a midwife if you so choose. In other words, midwifery is presented as a legal, not a health, issue.

Consumers Advocating the Legalization of Midwifery (CALM) clearly advocates the legalization of midwifery and fights to support both midwives and mothers-to-be.

▌What's Offered

For $25 you will get a subscription to CALM's quarterly newsletter on state legislative updates and help to fight for midwife legalization.

Friends of Homebirth
103 North Pearl Street
Big Sandy, TX 75755

Contact: Janet Tipton, Editor

▌Background

Most people assume that hospitals are not only the sole place to give birth, but that they provide the ultimate in care. Both assumptions are false.

An effective alternative successfully used by thousands of mothers every year is homebirth with the aid of a qualified midwife. Its safety? A recent study shows that infant mortality for midwives is one-third that of doctors delivering babies in a hospital. And care? An obstetrician may spend two to three hours on a delivery; the average midwife spends more than 30 hours.

Friends of Homebirth's mission is to make sure that natural childbirth at home with a midwife will remain an option for expecting parents.

▌What's Offered

A bimonthly newsletter, *Friends of Homebirth*, will keep you posted on the latest news on homebirth, provide you with valuable information in choosing a midwife, and keep you informed of current state and national laws and court rulings that affect your freedom of choice in childbirth. The newsletter has no price. If you find it of value, you are asked for a donation to defray printing and mailing costs.

Healthy Mothers, Healthy Babies
409 12th Street, SW
Washington, DC 20024-2188
202-638-5577

▌ Background

According to the Environmental Protection Agency, 20% of all pregnancies end in miscarriage. Cesarean births have inceased nearly tenfold. Malnutrition, and drug and alcohol abuse are more common in mothers-to-be than ever before. Yet, much of prenatal care is routine.

Healthy Mothers, Healthy Babies (HMHB) is a coalition of more than 90 organizations interested in maternal and infant health. By collaborative activities and the sharing of information and resources, they hope:

- ▪ To promote public awareness of preventive health habits for pregnant women
- ▪ To develop networks to share information among their member groups
- ▪ To distribute educational material to the general public
- ▪ To assist state and local groups.

▌ What's Offered

By contacting HMHB you will learn which national, state, or local organization can assist you. Its six-page, quarterly newsletter, *Healthy mothers, Healthy babies*, contains articles on the upcoming events and available health care information of other organizations and will be sent to you without charge.

Several low-cost products on maternal health and prenatal nutrition are also available.

Informed Homebirth/Informed Birth & Parenting
P.O. Box 3675
Ann Arbor, MI 48106
313-662-6857

▊ Background

Aside from giving birth with the assistance of a midwife, many pregnant women and fathers-to-be take separate birthing classes.

The Informed Homebirth/Informed Birth & Parenting is one of the four largest national organizations training childbirth educators in the United States.

▊ What's Offered

Training, consisting of workshops and seminars to become a certified childbirth educator and to gain the knowledge necessary to conduct workshops for parents, is available across the country and in home-study courses.

Referrals to a trained childbirth educator and a number of books on birthing and midwifery are also available.

International Childbirth Education Association
P.O. Box 20048
Minneapolis, MN 55420-0048
612-854-8660

▌ Background

There's more to natural childbirth than just using the services of a midwife or nurse-midwife.

The International Childbirth Education Association (ICEA) supports the concept of family-centered maternity care by:

- ▪ Emphasizing education and preparation for childbearing and breastfeeding
- ▪ Increasing the public's awareness of the latest findings relating to childbearing
- ▪ Encouraging individual care with minimal medical intervention
- ▪ Promoting the development and use of safe, low-cost alternatives in natural childbirth.

▌ What's Offered

Additionally, ICEA offers a program for the training of professional childbirth educators.

Membership ($20) for lay individuals includes a subscription to the 48-page quarterly, *International Journal of Childbirth Education*. It includes timely obstetrical and maternity care information, reviews of literature on childbearing, and regular features such as techniques for childbirth educators, a forum for administrators, and commentaries on a single topic.

For parents-to-be, new parents, and for anyone interested in or considering different alternatives in childbirth, the ICEA provides an extensive catalogue of many books, pamphlets, reprints, audio tapes, and videos on:

- Breastfeeding
- Pregnancy, birth, and childbirth preparation
- High-risk pregnancy
- Cesarean births
- Teenage pregnancy and outreach
- Grief and loss in pregnancy
- Parenting, careers, and pregnancy
- Parenthood and grandparenthood
- Infant, child care, and development
- Food and nutrition
- Health and family planning
- Midwifery.

Midwive's Alliance of North America
28 Galloway Road
Warwick, NY 10990
914-986-2995

Contact: Alice Sammon

▌ Background

Midwifery has a long and honored tradition in America. And, in spite of obstetricians and maternity hospitals, midwives are making a comeback.

The Midwive's Alliance of North America (MANA) is a professional organization of midwives, holding conferences and workshops and conducting advanced education classes for midwives.

▌ What's Offered

Many of MANA's practices involve alternative treatments such as visualization or guided imagery, therapeutic counseling, acupuncture, acupressure, and homeopathic medications.

A telephone call or letter will get any questions on midwifery answered and referrals to a midwife in your area.

NAPSAC
Route 1
P.O. Box 646
Marble Hill, MO 63764
314-238-2010

▌ Background

Much to most people's surprise, the incidence of problems associated with home birth and midwifery is far less than that of obstetricians and in hospitals.

NAPSAC stands for the National Association of Parents & Professionals for Safe Alternatives in Childbirth. It promotes home birth and midwifery as the safe alternative.

▌ What's Offered

More than just another professional organization of midwives, NAPSAC addresses all issues of birth and parenting. Holding conferences and workshops and conducting advanced education classes, NAPSAC's members receive continuing professional training in every aspect of child rearing. An example of a recent conference's topics other than midwifery and home birth were:

▪ Home schooling

- Natural birth after a cesarean
- Homeopathy
- Natural family planning
- The Brewer diet and gestational diabetes
- Full-time mothering.

A catalogue of material on pregnancy and childbirth, parenting, breastfeeding, and nutrition is available. An inquiry will get your questions about alternatives in childbirth answered and a referral to a midwife in your area.

National Association of Childbearing Centers
3123 Gottschal Road
Perkiomenville, PA 18074-9456
215-234-8068

▌ Background

Unlike the United States, in most places of the world children aren't born in hospitals. But in some places, including the United States, children are born in places for that very purpose. These special places are called birth centers.

Unlike hospitals, birth centers are not places to cure the sick. Rather, they provide programs for healthy, pregnant women and are places for their babies to be born. These programs and services include:

- Psychological counseling
- Pregnancy education
- Labor and birth support
- Information on infant care.

The purpose of the National Association of Childbearing Centers (NACC) is to develop quality childbearing facilities in the United States through the use of birth centers.

▌ What's Offered

Membership in NACC is normally open only to professionals in the field. Individual membership ($15) for the layperson is available and will entitle you to receive *NACC News*—a quarterly newsletter of birth center news and information, telephone counseling, and support through the Association's information network—and a membership directory listing all the birth centers in the United States.

National Network to Prevent Birth Defects
P.O. Box 15309
Southeast Station
Washington, DC 20003
202-543-5450

▌ Background

The goal of the National Network to Prevent Birth Defects (NNPBD) is to make potential parents, health care workers, and other interested individuals aware of the many hazards around us that lead to numerous birth defects.

▌ What's Offered

The group pays particular attention to excessive use of pesticides in food, toxic waste in our environment, drug and alcohol use by pregnant women, and better prenatal care. NNPBD supports a nation-wide network of state and local groups.

A quarterly ($20), 10-page newsletter reports on health and legislative news on birth defects. All articles have extensive medical journal references and are scholarly without being pedantic or jargon-filled. Some recent topics reported on have been:

- Groundwater pollution
- PCBs—how they affect the fetus
- Cocaine and pregnancy—addiction in the newborn
- Alcohol use during pregnancy.

The national group also sells a wide variety of pamphlets and books on related topics such as:

- Drinking water standards
- Benefits of breast milk
- Retardation
- Child abuse.

Positive Pregnancy & Parenting Fitness
51 Saltrock Road
Baltic, CT 06330
203-822-8573

▌ Background

Everyone can benefit from regular exercising, including mothers-to-be and newborn babies.

Positive Pregnancy & Parenting Fitness (PP&PF) focuses on pregnancy and parenting, but not from the viewpoint of birth. Rather, its philosophy is concerned with:

- Safe pregnancy, parenting, and baby exercising
- Stress management
- Relaxation, visualization, and coping skills
- Pregnancy and parenting information.

▍What's Offered

The PP&PF conducts pregnancy and parenting fitness instructor workshops and publishes a 16-page quarterly, *Positive Pregnancy & Parenting Fitness Newsletter*. Articles focus on only two areas:

- ▪ Regular features—recipes, upcoming workshops, news briefs, book reviews, and video reviews
- ▪ Relaxation/visual relaxation exercises.

PP&PF also publishes an extensive catalogue *Be Healthy*, offering books, audio tapes, videos, and many items for the newborn baby.

Read Natural Childbirth Foundation, Inc.
P.O. Box 956
San Rafael, CA 94915
415-456-8462

Contact: Margaret B. Farley, R.P.T.

▍Background

After decades of smaller families, single-parent families, and cohabitation pseudo-families, America seems once again to be going back to the traditional family—husband, wife, and children. More couples are having more children than in the last 25 years.

The Read Natural Childbirth Foundation, Inc. provides parents information about the Read Method of natural preparation for childbirth.

▌ What's Offered

The Read Method educates both the mother and father in a series of evening classes for the birth of the baby and includes information and training in:

- Nutrition and pregnancy
- Physiology and psychology of labor and birth
- Exercises for the expecting mother
- Relaxation techniques
- Breathing techniques for birthing
- Postpartum help.

The Foundation offers these classes in different areas of the country and sells several books and videos on the birthing experience.

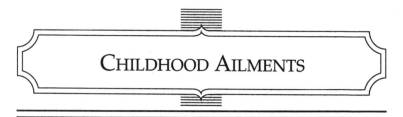

CHILDHOOD AILMENTS

American Sudden Infant Death Syndrome Institute
275 Carpenter Drive
Suite 100
Atlanta, GA 30328
800-232-SIDS
800-867-SIDS (in Georgia)

Contact: Sandy Brack, Vice President Development

■ Background

Close to 8000 healthy babies die each year without warning, without an apparent reason.

Sudden Infant Death Syndrome (SIDS), more commonly called crib death, is America's biggest killer of infants over the age of two weeks. Much confusion exists over SIDS, especially since it is not a disease. Rather, it is a classification of infant death when no other known cause is found.

The American Sudden Infant Death Syndrome Institute conducts research, provides clinical services, and fosters education for professionals on SIDS.

■ What's Offered

The Institute will provide you with information on SIDS, including statistical studies that help determine which mothers and babies are at greater risk.

Also available is information for health care professionals on testing infants for their risk of SIDS. This involves providing information on clinical services and diagnostic tests that can determine

SIDS risks. As an example of this research, it has been found that sleeping position—sleeping on the stomach aggravates the incidence of SIDS—is statistically significant.

Much of the available care for at-risk infants involves self-help, home care methods. The most common is the use of specially-developed SIDS monitors to be used when a baby is asleep.

Association of Birth Defect Children, Inc.
5400 Diplomat Circle
Suite 270
Orlando, FL 32810
407-629-1466

▌ Background

Recent studies indicate that more than 15% of American children are born with some type of birth defect; 250,000 of them are classified as major. Yet only 20% of the birth defects are genetic in origin. The remaining 80%, or 12% of all births, are the result of environmental agents.

The Association of Birth Defect Children (ABDC), Inc. acts as a clearinghouse to provide information about birth defects to parents and health care professionals.

▌ What's Offered

A $25 membership to ABDC entitles you to a subscription to their eight-page, quarterly newsletter that reports on new studies relating to the origin, prevention, and treatment of birth defects such as color and dyslexics, and immunotoxins. A regular parent's page presents news on other groups, upcoming regulations and laws, and short articles on a variety of maladies.

The Association also provides educational material about environmental agents associated with birth defects such as: drugs, chemicals, radiation, pesticides, alcohol, heavy metals, and so forth. ABDC also maintains a birth defect registry: an epidemiological forum to collect data about birth defects and environmental exposure.

They will answer requests for information about birth defects from anyone contacting them.

Child Health Alert
P.O. Box 338
Newton Highlands, MA 02161-9990

▮ Background

Caring for a child has never been easy. Today it seems far more complicated. Electric power lines, gas appliances, vitamins, junk food for kids, day care, TV, and on and on influence a child's life.

Child Health Alert is a four-page monthly ($18) newsletter concerned with reporting on what affects a child's health.

▮ What's Offered

Child Health Alert is certainly not an alternative health care journal; nonetheless, this newsletter contains much information that can be called complementary. Written by a team of physicians who specialize in pediatrics and child care, the articles have a doctor's seriousness and detail about them. Readers' queries are answered with the same thoroughness. Topics covered in the past include:

- Radon dangers for children
- Artificial sweeteners and children's health
- Sudden infant death and vaccinations

- Toy recalls
- Lyme disease and children
- Cough syrups and tranquilizers for children
- MSG and asthma in children.

All back issues are available and a sample copy will be sent on request.

Child Psychopharmacology Information Center
University of Wisconsin Department of Psychiatry
600 Highlan Avenue
Madison, WI 53792
608-263-6171

Background

It is now quite common for children to be on drugs. No, not the illegal kind we read about and see on TV, but pharmaceuticals prescribed for behavior problems. High jinks have been redefined to mean high crimes. Children are often put on these drugs by their schools to make them more manageable.

The Child Psychopharmacology Information Center serves as an information clearinghouse. More than 15,000 references from journals, books, government documents, seminar and meeting procedures, unpublished manuscripts, and reports are entered daily into a computerized database. Currently, topics referenced include:

- Psychiatric medication indications—children and adolescents
- Psychiatric medication safety—children and adolescents
- Child psychopharmacology research
- Innovative uses of psychiatric medications—children and adolescents

■ Psychiatric medication usage—special children and adolescents.

■ What's Offered

The University Center, although a nonprofit organization, charges a nominal fee for its computerized printouts consisting of bibliographies and copies of articles. In addition to this service, physician referral and support group lists are also available (although you should not count on their being alternative or even open to its suggestion).

A booklet entitled *Stimulants and Hyperactive Children: A Guide* is published under the University's auspices. It serves as a guide for patients, parents, and their families.

Children With Attention Deficit Disorders
499 NW 70th Avenue
Suite 308
Plantation, FL 33317
305-587-3700

Contact: Sandra F. Thompson, R.N.

■ Background

A common complaint is that people's attention span is growing shorter. Information comes to us in five-second TV spots, lest we turn the dial. Books, magazines, and newspapers have color pictures, charts, and diagrams, speaking clearly of their need to attract readers.

Amid all this, there are children who are suffering from a disease called attention deficit disorder (ADD). This ailment is more than not being able to focus on school work and not paying attention in class.

Some children are unable to sit still. Many cannot even remain seated. A few cannot wait their turn. Others blurt out answers to unasked questions. The symptoms go on. Many ADD children have more than one symptom—a few have all symptoms.

In response to the problem, Children With Attention Deficit Disorders, an organization of parents with children suffering from attention deficit disorders, was formed:

- To maintain support groups for parents of children with ADD
- To provide a forum for education of parents and health care professionals
- To act as a resource for information
- To assure that proper education is available to children with ADD.

▮ What's Offered

A $25 membership to ADD entitles you to three items: (1) a subscription to the monthly newsletter, *Chadder Box* containing news of upcoming events, book reviews, personal stories, and queries; (2) membership in a local support group and access to health care professionals specializing in ADD; and (3) the biannual *Chadder*, a 32-page magazine that contains articles on treatments, clinical studies, research reports, and information on support groups.

Exceptional Parent
Psy-Ed Corporation
1170 Commonwealth Avenue
Third Floor
Boston, MA 02134-4646
617-538-8961

▌ Background

A child's disability can devastate a family. As bad as that disability
or chronic ailment is, the effect it has on family members often
makes it worse.

Published eight times a year ($18), the four-color, nearly
100-page-long *Exceptional Parent* is devoted to disabled children
and their parents. It focuses on self-help, home-care, and bringing
disabled children into the mainstream of life.

▌ What's Offered

Exceptional Parent's regular features include family support and life
columns, medical and health news, and a fitness column. All of its
articles contain practical information and advice and stress the
positive—doing whatever you can with whatever you have. Recent topics have included:

- Grieving
- Social Security
- Advocacy
- Technology access
- Resources—selection criteria
- Outdoor activities
- Reviews of equipment for disabled children.

Feingold Association of the United States
P.O. Box 6550
Alexandria, VA 22306
703-768-FAUS

∎ Background

It is no secret that many children have learning disabilites; problems of behavior, health, and learning. Their names and symptoms are growing daily: hyperactivity, fidgetiness, excitability, impulsiveness, poor sleep habits, short attention span, inability to concentrate, compulsive aggression, self-mutilation, antisocial traits, irritability. The treatment of choice is drugs, often given without a parent's consent or even knowledge.

The Feingold Association of the United States (FAUS) believes that there is a better way, a way that they say has helped over 70% of children. That way is a specialized diet that completely eliminates synthetic food colors, flavors, and preservatives.

∎ What's Offered

The FAUS two-stage program of food elimination and then partial reintroduction is implemented by using the step-by-step guidelines in the *Feingold Handbook*. Additional books and pamphlets on which foods and medications must be eliminated and which ones may be reintroduced are also available. *Pure Facts*, published 10 times a year ($12), is a six-page newsletter filled with success stories, reader's letters, and short tidbits on news relating to the Feingold system. Recent articles have included the following topics:

- ∎ Ritalin safety—a drug routinely given to children with "behavior" problems
- ∎ New artificial sweeteners and FDA approval
- ∎ Behavior modification medication—report from medical experts.

National Committee for Prevention of Child Abuse
332 South Michigan Avenue
Suite 1600
Chicago, IL 60604-4357
312-663-3520

Contact: Diana Jemison

▮ Background

The purpose of the National Committee for Prevention of Child Abuse (NCPCA) is to present to the public a cornucopia of information resources—books, brochures, pamphlets, and videos—on child abuse in both English and Spanish in the hope that information will reduce its incidence. Additionally, it has several programs in prevention and public education, advocacy, and research and evaluation toward that end.

▮ What's Offered

NCPCA's catalogue contains many short, colorful booklets. The material is divided into four subjects: child abuse prevention, materials for parents, materials for children, and special subjects. A sample of brochure topics includes:

- ▮ Sexual abuse
- ▮ Physical abuse
- ▮ Emotional maltreatment
- ▮ Maltreatment
- ▮ Self-help
- ▮ Legal advice
- ▮ Teacher's and educator's guides.

National Information Center for Children
and Youth with Handicaps
P.O. Box 1492
Washington, DC 20013
800-999-5599
703-893-6061

▋ Background

Sympathy and empathy for a child with a handicap is all well and good, but getting information on helping the child do the best with what he or she has is more important.

The National Information Center for Children and Youth with Handicaps (NICCYH) is an information clearinghouse providing free material to parents, educators, health care professionals, advocates, and interested individuals on helping children with disabilities.

▋ What's Offered

Contact through their toll-free telephone number NICCYH will provide you with the following free material:

- Current information databases on disability topics
- Referrals to other organizations providing help
- Information packets on many disabilities
- Publications—*News Digest* three times a year (articles on current research) and *Transition Summary* once a year (current clinical practices and treatments)
- Technical assistance—workshops, seminars, and resource sharing.

Practical Allergy Research Foundation
P.O. Box 60
Buffalo, NY 14223
716-875-5578

█ Background

Allergic reactions—itchy eyes, raspy throat, runny nose—almost everyone seems to be allergic to something, especially children. Most people take an over-the-counter drug if they don't know what they're allergic to; others take something stronger from their doctor if the allergen has a name. But nothing seems to offer permanent relief.

The Practical Allergy Research Foundation (PARF) believes otherwise.

█ What's Offered

PARF, through Dr. Doris J. Rapp, a practicing allergist, has prepared a set of educational videos, audio tapes, and books that discuss unsuspected allergens: dust molds, pets, foods, and chemicals, as well as pollen.

Much of the material is devoted to childhood and infant allergies and their effect on learning and behavior. This very practical material will help you track down unsuspected allergens, discover the effect of allergens on your or your child's behavior, learn about childhood allergies and behavior problems such as learning deficits, and find out about environmental allergens in general.

Further Resources
see all resources under ORTHOMOLECULAR NUTRITION AND THERAPY
Autism Research Institute
College of Optometrists in Vision Development
Irlen Institute for Perceptual and Learning Development

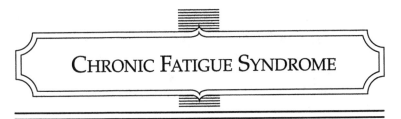

CHRONIC FATIGUE SYNDROME

CFIDS Association, Inc.
P.O. Box 220398
Charlotte, NC 28222-0398
704-362-CFID
704-365-9755 (fax)

▮ Background

Chronic Fatigue and Immune Dysfunction Syndrome (CFIDS) is characterized by an incapacitating fatigue and accompanying neurological problems. Accompanying symptoms can resemble other diseases, such as: mononucleosis, Lyme disease, lupus, and muliple sclerosis. Symptoms come and go over the months or years and, when flaring, are often completely debilitating.

The CFIDS Association's purpose is fourfold:

- Advocacy—insurance and disability
- Information—medical and clinical findings
- Research—case and demographic studies
- Education for CFIDS sufferers.

▮ What's Offered

A $25 membership includes a subscription to the quarterly *CFIDS Chronicle*, which has published close to 400 articles by experts from all over the world on a wide range of CFIDS-related topics. Regular features report current clinical research results, legal and insurance matters, coping, and news of local support groups. Feature articles over the years have included the following topics:

- Multitest CMI—diagnosis tool for CFIDS
- Interleukin-2
- CFIDS in children
- Acyclovir treatment—case study
- Stress and CFIDS
- Epstein Barr virus
- Treating CFIDS with Kutapressin™
- Insurance coverage
- AMA and CFIDS.

Several books and article reprints are also available. A national list of physicians and other health care professionals knowledgeable about CFIDS is maintained by local self-help groups.

Chronic Fatigue Immune Dysfunction Syndrome Society International
P.O. Box 230108
Portland, OR 97223
503-684-5261

▌ Background

The Chronic Fatigue Immune Dysfunction Syndrome Society (CFIDSS), International is a nonprofit, grass-roots organization that serves as a clearinghouse for chronic fatigue immune dysfunction syndrome information and patient support groups.

▌ What's Offered

Chronic fatigue syndrome—often called yuppie flu—is a feeling of fatigue that comes on suddenly and causes a debilitating, continuous tiredness that does not go away for several months or even years.

It's a rapidly spreading disease that orthodox medicine often denies by calling it psychosomatic or labels it as Epstein Barr virus with little clinical evidence. Nevertheless, no effective treatment—orthodox or alternative—now exists for all sufferers, although many patients have been helped by a wide variety of both orthodox and alternative therapies.

CFIDSS International publishes a newsletter, *The Reporter*, 10 times a year (included in their $20 yearly membership dues). Included in the newsletter are:

- CFIDS book reviews—extracts and summaries
- Local support group news—events and reader's tips
- Coverage of symposia—medical and patient groups
- Nutritional guidelines for CFIDS sufferers—from orthodox and alternative sources.

The organization also makes available many information packages on CFIDS, ongoing research results, and therapies, some of which are:

- Local support group lists
- Social Security—getting disability benefits
- Medical journal and magazine article reprints and abstracts.

Further Resources
Cancer Control Society
National Jewish Center For Immunology and Respiratory Medicine

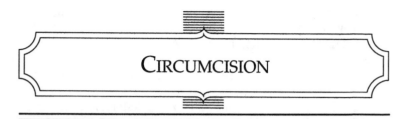

CIRCUMCISION

National Organization of Circumcision Resource Centers
P.O. Box 2512
San Anselma, CA 94960
415-488-9883

▮ Background

What's the most commonly performed surgery in the US? It's neither tonsillectomy nor heart surgery. It is circumcision.

The National Organization of Circumcision Resource Centers' purpose is to provide parents, health care professionals, and any concerned individual with medical and legal information on routine nonreligious and nonmedical circumcision. It believes that most of the reasons for circumcision are not only unnecessary but lead to medical problems specifically related to the practice.

▮ What's Offered

The organization's library, self education material, and telephone consultation are available. A video and several pamphlets on circumcision are offered for sale.

A quarterly ($15) four-page newsletter contains short articles on the medical implications of circumcision and updates on legal developments to stop its routine practice. Recent topics discussed have been on:

- Psychological motives behind physicians who perform the operation and parents who want it
- Urinary tract infections as a result of circumcision
- Female circumcision in America
- Legal news update.

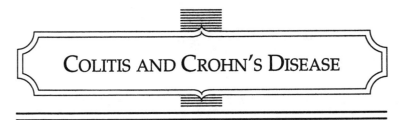

COLITIS AND CROHN'S DISEASE

Crohn's & Colitis Foundation of America, Inc.
444 Park Avenue South
New York, NY 10016-7374
800-343-3637
212-685-3440
212-779-4098 (fax)

Contact: Jane W. Present, National President

▌ Background

Two million men, women, and children suffer from Crohn's disease or inflammatory bowel disease (IBD). This year 30,000 more will be added to their ranks.

The Crohn's & Colitis Foundation of America (CCFA), Inc. is devoted to finding the cause and cure of colitis. Among their many research programs is one developing an animal model for Crohn's disease.

▌ What's Offered

The CCFA sponsors research through medical grants and serves as an educational service for patients, families, and physicians. A $25 annual membership includes the Foundation's newsletter, *Foundation Focus*, which reports on new treatments (orthodox as well as alternative), the research sponsored by the Foundation, and patients' comments. Additional publications include:

- *Treating IBD*
- *Crohn's Disease and Ulcerative Colitis Fact Book.*

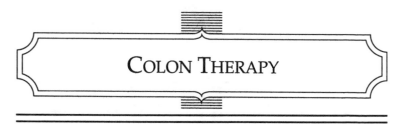

COLON THERAPY

California Colon Hygienists' Society
209 Morning Sun Avenue
Mill Valley, CA 94941
415-383-7224

Contact: Nancy Gardner, President

▌ Background

Each year almost 150,000 Americans are diagnosed as having colon or rectal cancer; 44% of them will die from it. In fact, colon cancer is the second leading cause of cancer deaths in the United States. Less deadly, but far more common are the millions of cases of colitis, diverticulitis, and other inflammatory bowel disorders. Yet most people are barely aware of the fact that somewhere in their body is a colon.

The colon is a tubular, hollow organ surrounding the outside wall of the abdomen. Digested food from the small intestine enters the colon in a liquid state where it is removed by muscular wave action.

However, due in part to the American diet of over-processed and over-cooked foods that leave a coating of slime on the colon's inner wall (resembling a coating of plaster on a wall), most people's colons resemble a cesspool. Accumulated and putrefying waste from decades ago may still be present.

The symptoms of a colon that, in non-medical terms, is toxic include every common complaint imaginable: extreme fatigue, trouble sleeping, overweight, muscle and joint pain, or colitis.

The California Colon Hygienists' Society (CCHS) is a professional organization of colon therapists.

▌ What's Offered

The best way to remove the wastes from the colon is through colonic irrigation, performed by a trained colon hygienist. Correct treatment involves more than just using water to flush out the wastes. Colon health is dependent upon pH—acid/alkaline balance—and many professionals encourage their clients to take mineral supplements and acidophilus (yogurt).

When seeking a professional, it is important to ask about his or her training and experience. Ask if other health care professionals refer patients to them, about the equipment (especially whether the machine has a disposable speculum and hoses), and what hygienic procedures are followed (everything not disposable should be sterilized).

The CCHS will provide you with a pamphlet on colonics and colon health and a referral to a therapist in your area.

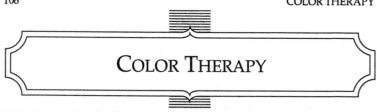

COLOR THERAPY

Dinshah Health Society
100 Dinshah Drive
Malaga, NJ 08328
609-692-4686

▌ Background

Everyone knows of the effect of light. Painters' studios always have
a north-light window so that their paintings look more lifelike.
Stage make-up is often applied under special full-spectrum lights
to look more real on the stage. The effect of moonlight on romance
is documented in thousands of love songs and poems.

But can light do more? Can it heal?

The Dinshah Health Society believes that it can and espouses
the therapeutic benefits of spectrochrome light (light mimicking
natural sunlight, also known as full spectrum light).

▌ What's Offered

Membership, just $3, includes a subscription to a *Breath Forecast* for
your area and their newsletter published twice a year. The Breath
Forecast involves light calculations based upon the new moon. The
newsletter has short abstracts on health matters (usually relating to
light) gleaned from many sources throughout the world. Recent
issues have discussed water fluoridation, additives in cigarettes,
and a decrease in learning disabilities in lime-green light.

Several books and pamphlets are sold on the health and
curative benfits of full-spectrum, natural light.

Further Resources
Irlen Institute for Perceptual and Learning Development

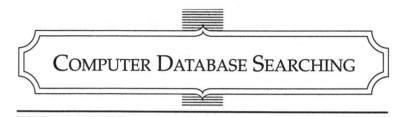

COMPUTER DATABASE SEARCHING

MEDLARS
MEDLARS Management Section
National Library of Medicine
8600 Rockville Place
Bethesda, MD 20894
800-638-8480
301-496-0822 (fax)

▌ Background

There are more than 3000 orthodox biomedical and health journals
regularly published. The National Library of Medicine not only
subscribes to all these journals; it places abstracts of every article
from every journal on a series of computer databases and makes
all this information available to everyone.

▌ What's Offered

By no means alternative or complementary, the information found
in MEDLARS contains the latest in conventional treatments and
new insights into the nature of almost every disease or ailment.
Additionally, every article on prevention, nutrition, and the use of
supplements written in mainstream medical and scientific journals
will also be found.

Seven regional medical libraries located at major medical
colleges can help you with your search request. Additionally,
many public libraries have access to the MEDLARS databases and
can perform the searches for you at a cost of between $10 and $50.

NAPRALERT
Program for Collaborative Research
in the Pharmaceutical Sciences
College of Pharmacy
University of Illinois at Chicago
P.O. Box 6998
Chicago, IL 60680
312-996-7253

▌ Background

It would be almost impossible for a nonresearcher to find scientific information about the therapeutic benefits of plants from scientific journals and books easily. About 200 journals and several thousand books in many languages would have to be looked at every month. To check that you hadn't missed anything it would also be necessary to search back to at least the 1960s.

NAPRALERT stands for NAtural PRoducts ALERT, a computer database of the scientific articles and books on the chemical constituents and pharmacology of plant, microbial, and marine animals that is available to anyone.

▌ What's Offered

Whether or not you have a computer, NAPRALERT is able to find medical information, results of biological tests, and chemical constituents of plant and marine animals from more than 75,000 scientific articles and books on natural products.

A $10 fee is charged for each computer search. Any information beyond three pages will cost you 50¢ a page.

Clearly, this is a useful service for practitioners and researchers. However, if you wish detailed scientific information about an herbal product or natural therapy, this computer search service may prove of value.

Further Resources
Herb Research Foundation

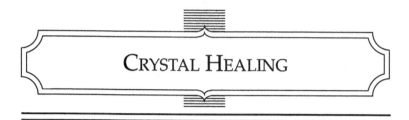

CRYSTAL HEALING

Lifespan Associates
70 Sable Court
Winter Springs, FL 32708
407-699-1672

Background

The New Age movement, along with Hamlet, believes that "there are more things in heaven and earth than are dreamt of in your philosophy." Among those new things are crystals, which are said to have the power to heal under certain conditions.

Lifespan Associates carries on the work of the late Dr. Marcel Vogel.

What's Offered

With the death of Vogel, much of the scientific and clinical research of the affects of crystals on the body, on compounds essential for life such as water, and on the therapeutic uses of crystals ended.

Aside from the metaphysical and psychological aspects of crystal therapy, research suggests that crystals have helped in substance abuse and trauma.

However, Lifespan Associates makes available all Vogel's works, including his audio tapes, videos, workbooks, back issues of the bimonthly *Psychic Research Newsletter*, specially cut meditation and healing crystals, and referrals to crystal therapy instructors.

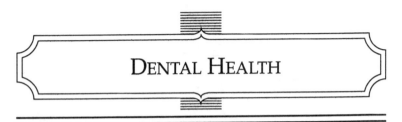

Dental Health

Environmental Dental Association
9974 Scripps Ranch Boulevard
Suite 36
San Diego, CA 92131
800-388-8124
619-586-7626

Contact: Giovanna DeSanti-Medina

▍Background

Mercury, a silvery looking, liquid metal, is the most toxic metal known to us—more toxic than arsenic. At room temperature it very slowly evaporates into the air.

If you're like most Americans, you have had a few cavities and your mouth contains several "silver" fillings. It is more than likely that these fillings are amalgam, a compound of 50% mercury and other metals.

The Environmental Dental Association (EDA) provides information to the general public on the health risks associated with mercury fillings and other hazardous dental procedures as well as the alternatives that are now available.

▍What's Offered

The EDA provides free information packets on amalgam fillings and the health risks associated with mercury toxicity. Their quarterly newsletter, *Informed Consent*, provides dentists with information on environmentally safe, nontoxic therapies. Also available are a number of books and audio tapes on mercury toxicity and other dental-related risks.

The EDA also maintains a referral service of more than 700 dentists and physicians concerned about the adverse effects of mercury and who treat ailments that may be related to them.

Holistic Dental Association
974 North 21st Street
Newark, OH 43055-2922
614-366-3309

▌Background

Although the mercury amalgam filling gets the most adverse publicity, other dental procedures may also prove harmful: surgery, periodontal treatment, implants, overuse of X-rays, TMJ, lack of preventive care.

The Holistic Dental Association (HDA), a professional organization of dentists, was formed to raise the standards of dental care and to disseminate information on safer, less toxic methods of dental care.

▌What's Offered

A bimonthly ($15) journal, *The Communicator*, provides the Association's members with technical articles on treatment techniques.

More important to the health care consumer, the HDA maintains a referral service of dentists who use a less invasive, more balanced approach to dental care.

Holistic Dental Digest

The Once Daily, Inc.
263 West End Avenue
Suite 2A
New York, NY 10023

▌ Background

Most people will do anything to avoid a visit to the dentist. Yet most adults have periodontal disease. False teeth are rampant among the middle-aged and elderly population. Crowns, caps, and fillings are nearly universal.

It's easy to go to the dentist after a problem occurs. But preventive dental information is harder to find.

▌ What's Offered

Dr. Jerry Mittelman, a practicing preventive, holistic dentist, publishes the four-page, bimonthly ($9.50) newsletter, *Holistic Dental Digest*. Its short and breezy articles written especially for the layperson will prove of use to anyone who still has and wants to keep his or her teeth for a lifetime. A sampling of article topics include:

- Bad teeth and heart attacks
- Home dental care devices—what to look for, how to use them
- TMJ—what it can do, how it happens, what can be done for it
- Plaque—what it is, what it does, what you can do about it
- Tooth clenching and astigmatism
- Teeth grinding—causes, dangers, cures
- Puffy gums—nutritional treatment.

International Academy of Oral Medicine and Toxicology
P.O. Box 17597
Colorado Springs, CO 80935-7597
719-599-8883
719-592-0436 (fax)

▌ Background

Many scientists believe that mercury fillings are so dangerous that they can often lead to learning deficits and delayed mental development in children and to infertility (one out of every five American couples is now infertile) and that they can be a causative factor in endometriosis, among other chronic conditions. They believe this in spite of protestations from the American Dental Association, and assurances from numerous and prestigious government and scientific panels disputing this claim.

The International Academy of Oral Medicine and Toxicology (IAMT), a professional organization of dentists and physicians, believes that the use of mercury in amalgam fillings may be one of the most serious health problems facing many Americans.

▌ What's Offered

Membership in the IAMT offers little to the average health care consumer. However, if you believe that mercury fillings may be a prominent cause of an illness affecting you or a family member, membership will provide you with a subscription to the Academy's monthly newsletter, *Bioprobe*, a review of the scientific literature and legislative activities in the area of mercury fillings.

Also available are several books on the dangers of mercury fillings and how to have them safely removed as well as information on how your dentist can test your reactions to the manmade materials in your mouth.

Additionally, a membership roster is available to help you find a dentist or physician in your area who is both knowledgeable about the problem and has had professional experience with it.

International Dental Health Foundation
11484 Washington Plaza West
Suite 307
Reston, VA 22090
703-471-83249

▮ Background

The International Dental Health Foundation (IDHF) is a professional organization of dentists and clinicians who use the Keyes system to treat periodontal diseases in a nonsurgical, conservative manner and then monitor the results microscopically.

The bases for the Keyes system of periodontal care are:

▮ Bacterial infections cause dental caries and destruction to the gum tissue
▮ Bacteria are contagious and can easily be transmitted between people
▮ Controlling bacteria can prevent and stop infection
▮ Conservative, noninvasive methods can be used to control these bacteria better than periodontal surgery.

In conjunction with the professional treatment, a self-care program that must be used daily is encouraged to prevent reinfection.

▮ What's Offered

An inquiry to the IDHF will bring you a copy of the Foundation's publication *Annotations*. A $10 annual membership fee will bring you three issues. A book, especially written for the layperson as a guide to self-care and professional dental treatment, *Second Opinion, Taking the Bite Out of Dentistry*, may also be ordered.

Included with this information will be a one- or two-page list of dentists in your state who use the Keyes System of preventive gum maintenance.

Further Resources
Association of Health Practitioners

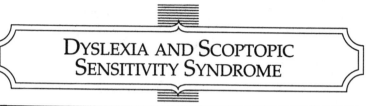

DYSLEXIA AND SCOPTOPIC SENSITIVITY SYNDROME

Irlen Institute for Perceptual and Learning Development
5380 Village Road
Long Beach, CA 90807
213-496-2550
213-429-8699 (fax)

Background

Scoptopic sensitivity syndrome (SSS) describes a group of visual perception dysfunctions affecting reading and writing. Its symptoms include light sensitivity; inability to distinguish the black-and-white contrast on a printed page; blurred, vibrating, or moving letters or words; loss of attention when reading; and an inability to judge distances.

A common name for one of the ailments is dyslexia, a reading disorder in which the letters of some words are rearranged.

Educational Psychologist Helen Irlen has developed a treatment for SSS and dyslexic dysfunctioning using color that is taught and practiced at the Irlen Institute for Perceptual and Learning Development.

What's Offered

Using colored plastic sheets and lenses, individualized prescription filters are developed for each patient. Interposing these sheets and lenses between the eyes and the page improve the ease and efficiency of reading. The technique can also improve patients with severe learning disabilities.

At present there are more than 40 clinics around the world where professionals trained by Irlen can diagnose and create the proper colored filters and lenses for the SSS sufferer.

If you contact the Institute, they will be happy to send you material on the therapy and refer you to a clinic in your area.

Orton Dyslexia Society
Chester Building
Suite 382
8600 LaSalle Road
Baltimore, MD 21204-6020
800-ABCD-123
410-296-0232
301-321-5069 (fax)

▋ Background

Dyslexia is not a disease of intelligence; many dyslexics are of superior intelligence. Dyslexia is a disease involving language; dyslexics have trouble mastering language skills, especially reading.

The Orton Dyslexia Society, a nonprofit organization providing educational information and material for the general public and undertaking and reporting medical research to health care professionals, is the country's oldest organization devoted to dyslexia.

▋ What's Offered

Membership, $50 for individuals and $90 for families, includes:

- Affiliation with a local support group
- Current educational and research findings on dyslexia

- Publication discounts
- Help in finding and evaluating a treatment program
- Subscriptions to their quarterly newsletter, *Perspectives on Dyslexia* and the yearly *Annals of Dyslexia.*

Much of the information in the Society's newsletter is directed toward physicians and educators, but enough is written for parents for it to be considered. Some topics covered include:

- Adult dyslexics
- Gender differences among dyslexics
- Language development in children
- Parental coping
- Adapting for college preparedness
- Self-esteem in dyslexics.

The Society's toll-free hotline will also answer any general and personal questions about dyslexia and help you find special education for dyslectic children.

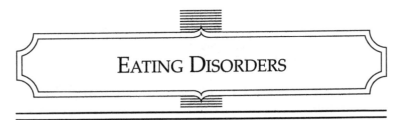

EATING DISORDERS

American Anorexia/Bulimia Association, Inc.
418 East 76th Street
New York, NY 10021
212-734-1114

Contact: Ann Meyers, Assistant Director

▌Background

To someone with an eating disorder, food is used neither for nutrition nor pleasure but as a psychological means of avoiding painful thoughts and feelings. Two common ailments are anorexia and bulimia. Anorexics starve themselves; Bulimics obsessionally overeat and then vomit.

The American Anorexia/Bulimia Association (AABA), Inc. believes that eating disorders are psychological problems that require psychological counseling.

▌What's Offered

A $50 yearly membership to AABA includes an extensive reading list, a subscription to their quarterly newsletter *AABA*, and a referral service to self-help groups, other organizations, treatment centers, and individual health care professionals. Some recent topics in the newsletter have included:

- Eating disorders and problems of relationships
- Prozac as a treatment option
- Sports and exercising for eating disorder sufferers
- Danger signs to watch for in anorexia and bulimia.

Anorexia Nervosa and Related Eating Disorders, Inc.
ANRED
P.O. Box 502
Eugene, OR 97405
503-344-1144

Contact: Dr. Jean Rabel

▌ Background

We live in a society that promotes a cultural ideal of a perfect body that should be the goal of all, especially for women. That ideal, rather than being based upon a goal of optimal health, conforms to one particular view of physical beauty. Many people accept this, believing that by looking like a certain model or having the physical competence of a certain professional athlete, they will achieve the happiness they so desperately seek. Such a decision makes them vulnerable to eating and exercise disorders.

The Anorexia Nervosa and Related Eating Disorders (ANRED), Inc., formed several years ago to study these ailments, also:

- Collects information about eating and exercise disorders
- Forms and promotes the formation of self-help groups
- Provides training to health care professionals who work with eating and exercise disorder patients
- Speaks out and educates the general public about these ailments.

▌ What's Offered

ANRED publishes a variety of booklets on anorexia nervosa, bulimia, compulsive eating, and compulsive exercising along with a 10-issue ($10) per year newsletter, *ANRED Alert*. All the material is presented in a no-nonsense style that cuts through much of the scientific language and theory. Much of the information is gathered both from the scientific literature and from the many self-help and support groups that deal with these illnesses.

Bulimia Anorexia Self Help, Inc.
Deaconess Medical Office Center
6125 Clayton Avenue
Suite 215
St. Louis, MO 63139
800-762-3334
314-768-3794 (fax)

▋ Background

Many persons believe that eating disorders require professional health care in a clinical setting. Bulimia Anorexia Self Help (BASH), Inc. operates such a clinic. But, BASH also publishes many monographs and a magazine on anorexia nervosa and bulimia that discuss a variety of self-help and alternative approaches.

▋ What's Offered

Their monthly ($25) *BASH Magazine* contains scientific articles for health care professionals on eating disorders, book reviews, and digests of scientific periodical articles relating to eating disorders. Article topics in the past have included:

- Food allergy influences
- Psychiatric profiles of those with eating disorders—binge eating, excessive thinness
- Group therapy
- Spiritual guidance as a part of therapy
- Self-starvation—damage to bone structure
- Eating disorders and mood disorders.

Help Anorexia & Bulimia, Inc.
P.O. Box 2992
Culver City, CA 90231-2992
213-558-0444

▮ Background

Like other organizations devoted to eating disorders, Help Anorexia & Bulimia, Inc. offers similar services. Unlike them however, this goup was founded by an individual indirectly affected by the problem. It now boasts an advisory board of distinguished specialists in the field.

▮ What's Offered

Contacting Help Anorexia & Bulimia will bring you a bulletin of the services they provide and a reading list for follow-up information. Some of those services, all of which are available at no charge, include:

- Education—seminars, discussion groups, and support groups
- Referrals—physicians, psychological professionals
- Information—reading lists
- Crisis assistance—one-on-one help in coping
- Research referrals—abstracts, bibliographies, monographs, and books.

Always on the lookout to further what they already do, a newsletter is in the offing.

National Anorexic Aid Society
5796 Karl Road
Columbus, OH 43229
614-436-1112

▌ Background

The National Anorexic Aid Society (NAAS) was formed to offer help to people suffering from the eating disorders of anorexia nervosa, bulimia nervosa, and other related ailments. Their primary goal is to provide education and treatment.

▌ What's Offered

A $20 membership to NAAS will bring you the following four benefits:

- Quarterly newsletter and bibliography of current research and findings
- An international referral list of health care professionals and support groups
- Audio tapes of past workshops on eating disorders
- National hotline to answer questions and locate treatment centers, practitioners, and support groups.

National Association of Anorexia Nervosa and Associated Disorders
ANAD
P.O. Box 7
Highland Park, IL 60035
312-831-3438

▌ Background

No one can argue against being slim and trim as an adjunct to good health. But starving yourself for perceived aesthetic reasons is not a part of anyone's health regimen, only a beauty one. Whatever their causes, cycles of starving and gorging by young women is neither normal nor part of a search for health. Rather, it is a recognized disease.

The National Association of Anorexia Nervosa and Associated Disorders (ANAD) is an educational and self-help organization dedicated to alleviating eating disorders.

▌ What's Offered

Composed primarily of anorexics and their families, ANAD offers:

- Counseling to patients and their families
- Referral list of more than 3000 therapists, hospitals, and clinics in the United States and Canada
- Information and bibliographies to health professionals and interested people
- Self-help groups and local chapters
- Research—over 1400 patient studies
- Patient advocacy—insurance and consumer products.

A $15 membership entitles you to a monthly, four-page newsletter and membership in a local, self-help support group. The newsletter contains stories of eating disorder sufferers and how they have coped, treatment modalities, up-beat editorials, and local group news.

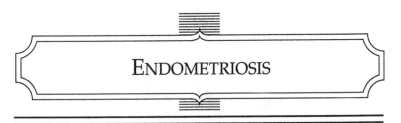

ENDOMETRIOSIS

Endometriosis Association
8585 North 76th Place
Milwaukee, WI 53223
800-992-ENDO
414-355-2200

Contact: Joan D. Lawrence

▮ Background

Endometriosis is a disease affecting five million women in America between the ages of 11 and 50. It comes from the word *endometrium*, the tissue lining the inside of the uterus. This uterine tissue builds up each month and is then shed during the menstrual cycle. In women with endometriosis, the tissue is found outside the uterus.

The Endometriosis Association is an international self-help organization of women with endometriosis and interested indivduals that offers:

- Local chapters and support groups
- Medical research and data registry
- Fact sheets, pamphlets, and brochures
- Newsletter
- Education programs
- Information clearinghouse
- Technical assistance.

▌ What's Offered

A yearly $25 membership fee includes their bimonthly newsletter whose articles have included information about:

- Intestinal problems
- Knowing what's in your medical records
- Adhesions due to active endometriosis and surgery
- Hysterectomies for women with endometriosis
- Research findings from symposia and conferences
- Synarel—the first GnRH- (gonadatropic-releasing hormone) approved drug.

If you would like further information, a referral to a health care professional in your area, or a basic information kit for $3.75 if you suspect you may have endometriosis, telephone or write.

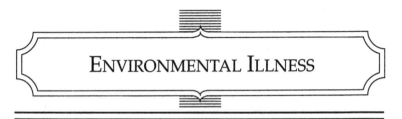

ENVIRONMENTAL ILLNESS

American Environmental Health Foundation
8345 Walnut Hill Lane
Suite 200
Dallas, TX 75231
214-361-9515

▌ Background

As our environment rapidly changes from a completely natural one to an artificial world, more and more people are finding their health adversely affected by it. Everything from headaches, sniffles, and skin problems to life-threatening ailments brought on by exposure to toxic pollutants are reported.

The American Environmental Health Foundation (AEHF), a non-profit foundation engaged in original research in environmental diseases, has four stated purposes for its existence:

- ▪ To support and conduct medical research in environmental health
- ▪ To disseminate information on environmental health to professionals and the general public
- ▪ To provide environmentally safe products
- ▪ To support education and training of professionals.

▌ What's Offered

Membership ($15) entitles you to a subscription to the *AEHF Newsletter.* In it you will find information on current research in environmental illness and practical suggestions for the afflicted. Other publications are in the form of books, reports, articles, and audio cassettes on environmentally triggered disorders, some technical and intended for the professional but many written for the general public.

A wide variety of unusual products such as pollutant-detection kits; medical supplies; and nontoxic, personal hygiene, cleaning, and filtration products—all especially designed for chemically sensitive people—are also available.

The AEHF also conducts several technical conferences a year for professional health care practitioners.

American Institute of Biomedical Climatology
1023 Welsh Road
Philadelphia, PA 19115
215-673-8368

▌ Background

Weather affects health. Everyone living in Los Angeles knows that when the Santa Ana winds blow in from the desert, people are more on edge and the city's homicide rate soars. This is weather that Raymond Chandler called "breadknife weather," when a wife looked fondly at the back of her husband's neck while slicing bread for dinner. The Levant in the Middle East and the Scirocco in Africa have the same effect. The depleting ozone layer may be the major cause of rising skin cancer rates. On the other hand, research confirms the beneficial effects of negative ions in the air; don't we all feel better near running water and when we're at the beach?

The American Institute of Biomedical Climatology (AIBC) acts as a clearinghouse for information on the effects of climate (outdoor and indoor) on health.

▌ What's Offered

A $25 membership to AIBC entitles you to receive the Institute's bimonthly *AIBC News Bulletin*. Each issue has one or two paragraph articles summarizing various sources where readers may get more information on many of the more common environmental factors affecting health such as electric fields, air pollution, ozone layer depletion, and indoor environments.

Earthwise Consumer
P.O. Box 1506
Mill Valley, CA 94942
415-383-5892

▌ Background

While "the environment" may merely be the latest *cause célèbre* in a long list, personal environmental health must be a matter of concern for everyone.

Earthwise Consumer, published eight times a year ($20), is primarily concerned with the safety and efficacy of the products you buy for yourself and your house.

▌ What's Offered

What you will find in this pleasant little newsletter is a review of products you use (or should use) every day. It identifies and differentiates product characteristics from a personal and planetary environmental standpoint. In other words, it is less concerned with the efficiency of the product than with its effect on you and your environment.

Products are rated on a 12-point scale from nontoxic to socially conscious business practices. Whatever your politics and environmental views, using natural alternative products that do no harm and work well may very well do less harm. Regular newsletter features include: letters to the editor, readers' tips, product and book reviews, and environmental news. Article topics discussed in recent issues are:

- Choosing "green" products
- Organic skin-care products
- Buying and using recycled products
- Toxic carpet alternatives.

Several books on maintaining a safer personal environment are also available.

Environmental Health Network
P.O. Box 1628
Harvey, LA 70058
504-362-6574

Contact: Linda King, Director

Background

It is difficult to find a source of information on environmental illnesses that satisfies both health care professionals and patients alike. Information is either so technical that it is useless to all but a specialist or is so watered down that practitioners refuse to even look at it. Even worse, it is often the professional who cannot find a laboratory to perform the tests needed or a company selling products to help his or her patients.

The Environmental Health Network (EHN) bridges that gap.

▌ What's Offered

The EHN, through the information it provides, empowers both groups by:

- ▪ Providing practical information to patients and health care practitioners
- ▪ Networking health care professionals with people exposed to toxins
- ▪ Sponsoring conferences on environmental health.

A $15 membership entitles you to the Network's quarterly, *Profiles on Environmental Health.* In it you will find technical articles on toxic contamination and the ailments they cause. Aside from the articles there are excerpts from other publications, letters to the editor, readers' surveys, upcoming events, and lists of books and other resources. You do not need extensive scientific knowledge to understand and benefit from the information, but you do have to have some fundamental grounding in the basics. All articles are thoroughly researched, cover both toxins and patient symptoms, and have references for follow-up research. Some recent topics include:

- ▪ Toxic contamination and stress
- ▪ Poverty and pollution
- ▪ Manganese—alloys and compounds
- ▪ Potassium permanganate
- ▪ Fashion chemical hazards.

The EHN also provides a physician referral service to those who believe that they may have been exposed to environmental toxins.

Environmental Health Watch
4115 Bridge Avenue
Cleveland, OH 44113
800-222-9348
216-961-4646

▌ Background

The Environmental Health Watch (EHW) is solely involved with educating the public about indoor pollution and environmental concerns.

Some of the concerns in this area are:

- Water conservation and filtration
- Nontoxic material utilization
- Biodegradable products
- Heating, air conditioning, and ventilation
- Inspection for health hazards
- Radon testing and treatment
- Air cleaning for health.

▌ What's Offered

The EHW conducts seminars and workshops for professionals, such as environmental consultants, manufacturers of "green" products, architects, and contractors. It is a prime source for locating someone qualified to deal with indoor pollution problems or new construction.

If you are contemplating a major construction project (even a new home), you may wish to attend one of their conferences. Not only will you learn from the speakers, but the exhibitors and attendees will give you product and service information and many contacts.

Associated with EHW is the Housing Resource Center at 1820 West 48th Street, Cleveland, OH 44102 (216-281-4663).

EHW's monthly newsletter, *Your Home,* will answer many common concerns about indoor pollution, provide you with a list of upcoming workshops, and review new products. Their illustrated quarterly, *Housemending Resources,* is devoted to a single topic such as remodeling, home heating systems, or basement water problems.

The Housing Resource Center publishes *Blueprint for a Healthy House,* a national directory of indoor pollution resources of products, publications, professional services, materials, and other information for consumers.

Books and audio tapes on making your house safer or building a healthy one are offered for sale.

Greenkeeping
Greenkeeping, Inc.
P.O. Box 28
Annandale-on-Hudson, NY 12504
914-246-6948
914-246-5243 (fax)

▌ Background

Many people would like to buy environmentally safe and healthy products. Many, like the rest of us, are inundated with catalogues promising that their products are as "green" as grass. Few of these catalogues are aware of the tests done on these products; less are aware that tests should be done.

But *Greenkeeping,* a bimonthly ($22.50), 30-odd-page magazine is not just another catalogue—in fact, it's not a catalogue at all—touting "green" products.

▌ What's Offered

What you will find are detailed reviews of products and alternative suggestions for using many of the products you now use.

For example, a recent issue had an article on alternatives to lead-acid and alkaline batteries for small appliances and included resources where you can buy them. Another article discussed hair dyes. At first thought, this seemed a rather benign and boring issue. But the article went on to point out that all FDA-certified dyes contain some lead and possibly arsenic, many as much as 10 parts per million. Included with the article were several reviews for hair colorings. Each review listed the ingredients and specified whether they were organically grown.

Still another article covered chemicals in the school—maintenance, janitorial supplies, and schoolroom supplies. The article gave alternative sources for all these and even mentioned several sources for certified nontoxic art supplies.

You get the picture. If you want to know more about products that are safe for the environment and yourself, consider a sample copy for $3.

Human Ecology Action League
P.O. Box 49126
Atlanta, GA 30359-1126
404-248-1898

▌ Background

As more and more chemicals are being used, more and more people are finding themselves sensitive to more and more of them. In fact, ecological illness: muliple chemical sensitivity is called the twentieth century illness.

The Human Ecology Action League (HEAL) was founded to help those with environmental illness (EI) to live happy and fulfilling lives in spite of their sensitivities to common household and industrial products. HEAL's goals are:

- To increase awareness of environmental conditions affecting health
- To serve as an information clearinghouse on known chemicals causing sensitivities
- To minimize use of pesticides and other toxic chemicals
- To encourage research in chemical sensitivities
- To establish local self-help and support groups for the chemically sensitive.

What's Offered

A $20 membership will get you HEAL's quarterly, *The Human Ecologist*. Its regular features include letters to the editor and readers' tips, a resource bulletin board, environmental health news, pesticide update, and book reviews.

Many articles are first-person experiences of those with EI. Others are practical and informative with tips and guidelines for specific problems. Along with their references those articles have something a little extra: an abstract of the article to help you decide if it warrants your reading. Topics covered in the past have included:

- Coping with emotional stress of EI
- Migraine headaches and pollution
- Workers' illnesses—diseases of advanced technology
- Benefits of germanium for those with EI
- Intestinal parasites
- Dangers of formaldehyde
- Plants that clean the air.

National Center for Environmental Health Strategies
1100 Rural Avenue
Voorhees, NJ 08043
609-429-5358

Contact: Mary Lamielle

▌ Background

Some chemicals bother everyone. Some chemicals bother no one. But people suffering from asthma, allergies, various breathing and lung ailments, and multiple chemical sensitivities experience slight to debilitating reactions to one or more chemicals. The three groups of people at greatest risk to chemicals are industrial workers, occupants of buildings without air exchanges, and people continually exposed to the same chemicals.

The National Center for Environmental Health Strategies (NCEHS) provides technical and educational information; legal advocacy services, and referrals in the area of chemical sensitivity and related health issues.

▌ What's Offered

NCEHS' $15 annual membership entitles you to their quarterly newsletter, *The Delicate Balance*. The articles are wide-ranging, professionally done, and informative. Some sample topics from a recent issue include:

- ▌ Update on pending legislation
- ▌ Nitrous oxide toxicity
- ▌ Air quality inside moving automobiles
- ▌ Methylene chlorine outgassing
- ▌ Indoor Air Quality Act
- ▌ Legislative news
- ▌ Environmental studies
- ▌ Electromagnetic health risks

▪ Chemically sensitive patients
▪ Killing pests with heat.

National Foundation for the Chemically Hypersensitive
P.O. Box 9
Wrightsville, NC 28480-0009
517-697-3989

▍Background

Fundamentally, people are as diiferent as fingerprints. We all know people who seem to exist on junk food and behave like couch potatoes throughout a long, apparently healthy life. Others restrict their food to only the healthiest and vigorously exercise daily, yet die in midlife. Still others are sensitive to the point of debilitation from chemicals that the rest of us find, at worst, only annoying.

The National Foundation for the Chemically Hypersensitive (NFCH) is dedicated to serving those who are highly sensitive to our modern environment.

▍What's Offered

A $10 membership to NFCH will entitle you to a great deal:

▪ Counseling
▪ Referrals to several doctors in your area who specialize in environmental illnesses
▪ Make available a reading list on environmental illnesses
▪ Put you in contact with a local support group or help you to form one
▪ Help you toward a healthier lifestyle
▪ Take your history and add it to their computerized database

■ Offer one of their members to act in a one-on-one relationship with you

■ Assist you with chemical sensitivity and dietary problems.

A newsletter ($10) will soon be available and will provide additional information on multiple chemical sensitivities, environmental illness, food intolerance, total allergy syndrome, candida, and chronic fatigue.

Society for the Study of Biochemical Intolerance
1675 North Freedom Boulevard
Suite 11-E
Provo, UT 84604
801-373-8500

■ Background

There are many proposed theories of chemical sensitivity—from completely psychological to chemical toxin exposures.

The Society for the Study of Biochemical Intolerance (SSBI) encourages the study of the adverse reactions people have to aromatic and similar chemical constituents.

These chemicals form a broad group called phenolics. Research indicates that they play a major role in allergies, hypersensitivities, intolerances, and imbalances, especially to those people who suffer from chemical sensitivities in general, behavior and learning disorders, and chronic degenerative diseases.

■ What's Offered

The SSBI seeks to further this research, much of which was developed by Dr. Robert W. Gardner at Brigham Young University. Its members, mainly scientists, researchers, and allergists, use

Gardner's techniques for treating chemical sensitivities and help patients adapt to the environment in which they find themselves, of necessity, a part.

Wary Canary
Wary Canary Press
Box 2204
Boulder, CO 80522
303-224-0083

▌ Background

When miners went down into the pits they would take canaries with them. Canaries, very sensitive to chemicals in the air including the gases given off in the mines, would die before the miners were even aware of a problem. When their chirping stopped the miners knew that they had better get out of the mine fast!

There are people who are chemically sensitive to the polluting gases in the air and suffer from environmental illness (EI). Perhaps they, too, are acting as canaries for the rest of us, sending a warning to us all that the air we breathe and the food we eat may soon not be able to support life.

While warning the world of possible ecological disaster is a worthy undertaking, people who suffer from EI will be the ones who most immediately benefit from *Wary Canary*, a 16-page quarterly ($15).

▌ What's Offered

Wary Canary's articles run no more than a page or two and offer specific, practical advice followed by a list of several resources one can go to for further help. Regular features include readers' letters and a bulletin board of news of other groups. Articles from the first few issues have included information on:

- Exercise and the chemically sensitive
- EPA neuropsychological study on pesticides
- Gluten intolerance and Alzheimer's disease
- Meditation and longevity
- Relocation and health
- Clinical ecology and EI patients.

Further Resources
> see all resources under ORTHOMOLECULAR NUTRITION AND THERAPY
> Allergy Information Association
> American Academy of Environmental Medicine
> *Environmental Nutrition*
> Enviro-Tech Products
> Practical Allergy Research Foundation

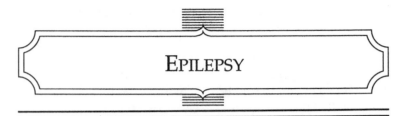

Epilepsy Foundation of America
4351 Garden City Drive
Landover, MD 20785
800-EFA-1000 (information and referrals)
301-459-3700

Background

We are as much bioelectric beings as biochemical ones. Many ailments result from imbalances in the body's electric functioning. Such is the case with epilepsy, a chronic condition caused by changes in the electrical function of the brain and characterized by seizures.

The Epilepsy Foundation of America (EFA) is dedicated to the welfare of people with epilepsy while it:

- Supports research to develop better treatments
- Provides information and education to the public
- Acts as an advocacy organization to fight discrimination against epileptics.

What's Offered

Joining the EFA ($15) will automatically make you a member of one of their local self-help groups and give you a subscription to the EFA's monthly, 12-page newsletter, *National Spokesman*.

Local groups for epileptics and their families will:

- Provide information for families
- Offer a local referral service

- Act as a support organization and an advocate for those being discriminated against
- Help find employment and employee education
- Organize recreational activities for youngsters with epilepsy.

Many pamphlets, books, brochures, bulletins to be distributed at schools, films, audio tapes and videos pertaining to epilepsy (some in Spanish as well as English) are also available.

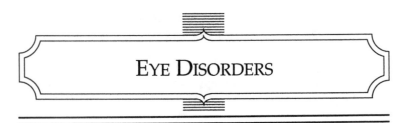

EYE DISORDERS

Bio-Zoe, Inc.
P.O. Box 49
Waynesville, NC 28786
800-426-7581
704-452-0472

▌ Background

Glaucoma, macular degeneration, cataracts, subconjunctoval hemorrhage—all are ailments affecting the eyes and resulting in a loss of vision.

Gary Price Todd, M.D., is one of the country's leading specialists in the treatment of eye disorders, specializing in the use of nutrition and lifestyle changes.

▌ What's Offered

Besides his clinical practice, Todd also makes available much of the material he has written, audio tapes of the lectures he has given, and nutrients he has prescribed for his patients, through Bio-Zoe.

Available as well are summary sheets on various conditions affecting eyes and vision. Each one has a summary of the ailment along with the nutritional and lifestyle changes that have been shown to help.

Bio-Zoe also sells specially developed nutritional products and several books on alternative approaches to treating and preventing some common, but major, diseases.

College of Optometrists in Vision Development
Box 285
Chula Vista, CA 91912
619-425-6191

▌ Background

Seeing is believing, but it's also inspecting, identifying, and inter-
preting all that surrounds us. While our ancestors needed their eyes
for hunting and farming, the reliance on eyesight for close, sus-
tained work has never been greater.

Even with "20/20 eyesight" you may have difficulties related
to working at close distances. The term itself is misleading. It does
not mean that you have "perfect" vision; only that you can see well
at distances of 20 feet or more. It does not refer to how well you see
at 12 to 16", the distance most of us need at work or school. The
stress that close work places on the eyes can cause headaches;
blurred vision; tired, itchy, or watery eyes; or a variety of vision-
related problems. Some estimates state that between 6 to 15 million
Americans suffer some form of eye problems on a regular basis:
including the inability to properly focus, aim the eye, binocular
vision problems, visual movement and blurring, and visual-per-
ceptual difficulties.

A form of treatment that does not rely on eyeglasses or
surgery has emerged in the past few years. It is known as vision
therapy or behavioral optometry. Vision therapy, however, relates
to more than eyesight. These problems are often mis-diagnosed as
learning disabled or dysfunctional, especially in children. Several
important studies have shown that it has remarkable success with
children diagnosed as learning disabled (73% improvement) or
having trouble in school (25% improvement).

The College of Optometrists in Vision Development (COVD)
is an international certifying organization for optometrists who
specialize in vision therapy.

▌ What's Offered

Membership in College is open only to professional optometrists trained in vision therapy, and its periodicals and other publications are only suitable for professionals in the field.

But the COVD will be happy to provide you with several explanatory pamphlets on vision therapy and refer you to an optometrist who is a member in your area.

For more detailed information about vision therapy, including a catalogue of pamphlets for the general public, books for professionals and interested individuals, software, training material, audio tapes and videos (many of which are for parents of children with vision or learning problems, and the adult with similar problems), contact:

Optometric Extension Program Foundation
2912 South Daimler Street
Santa Ana, CA 92705-5811
714-250-0846

International Myopia Prevention Association
R.D. 5, Box 171
Ligonier, PA 15658
412-238-2101

Contact: Donald Rehm

▌ Background

One-third of all schoolchildren born with normal vision become nearsighted during their school years. Many of them have vision that has deteriorated so badly that they are legally blind without their glasses. Modern ophthamology ignores much of modern research that disputes the stated claim that the condition is due entirely to heredity.

For example, monkeys with eyes nearly identical to humans develop myopia under certain scientifically controlled situations. Navy submarine personnel working in a visually confining environment develop myopia faster than other personnel. Sixty percent of Eskimo schoolchildren are myopic even though almost none of their parents and grandparents suffered from it.

The International Myopia Prevention Association believes that myopia is a disease of civilization caused by excessive reading and close work.

What's Offered

Finding that people with myopia have eyes that measure 25% longer than normal, the Association believes that wearing stronger and stronger eyeglasses as time goes on causes vision to deteriorate faster than if no eyeglasses were ever worn.

The Association makes available a book on myopia that not only explains it fully but will give you some preventive tips when doing close work.

They also prepare special "myopter" viewers to replace glasses. They believe that using this viewer will fool the eyes into believing that they are looking into the distance while doing close work and eliminate the stress on the eyes. The resulting lower stress is said to reduce the myopia and prevent further deterioration.

National Eye Research Foundation
910 Skokie Boulevard
Suite 207A
Northbrook, IL 60062
800-621-2258

Contact: Pamela A. Baker, Executive Director

▌ Background

Ask any group of people to select the most important of their senses: seeing, hearing, tasting, smelling, and touching. Odds are that every one of them will say that their sight is the most important. In spite of that, how many of us take as much care of our eyes as we do our hair or fingernails?

The National Eye Research Foundation (NERF) serves not only as a professional organization of eye care specialists and researchers, but acts to support vision research, to certify eye care assistants, to set standards for eye care products, to publish research findings and case studies, and to serve as an advocate for the public's concern in eye care matters.

▌ What's Offered

The Foundation's publications and educational facilities serve only professionals. A specially prepared *Patient Newsletter* is sent to members for their patients and contains current eye and health care articles.

However, NERF's technical staff will answer any of your questions about eye care and contact lenses and provide either you or your doctor with referrals to eye care specialists in your area of the country.

Further Resources
> see all resources under NUTRITION AND DIET
> see all resources under ORTHOMOLECULAR NUTRITION AND THERAPY

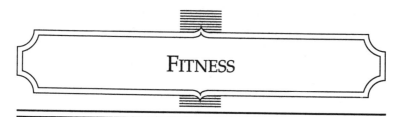

FITNESS

American Running & Fitness Association
9310 Old Georgetown Road
Bethesda, MD 20814
301-897-0197

Contact: Lisa Gundling, Public Information Specialist

▌ Background

Exercise may be at least as important to health and longevity as diet. It may turn out to be more important. Although the food you eat is the fuel your body needs to keep you healthy, exercising your heart and other muscles is what keeps them functioning at peak performance.

Whether for health reasons or reasons of vanity, many people are exercising. Because so few of us take exercise training seriously, sports-related injuries are on the rise.

The American Running & Fitness Association (AR&FA), an organization of athletes and sports medicine professionals, was formed to educate the public about the health benefits of regular aerobic exercise.

▌ What's Offered

A $25 membership to AR&FA entitles you to a subscription to the Association's eight-page, monthly newsletter, *Running & FitNews*. In addition to readers' queries with answers from experts, its short abstracts taken from health and medical journals keep readers up to date on any information related to sports and health. Recent article topics have included:

- Fluid intake to improve athletic performance
- Carbohydrate loading—speed versus distance
- Cookware—safety
- Exercise drinks—correct use
- Exercise for pregnant women—effect on unborn
- Training—guided imagery.

Just a few additional benefits of membership are:

- Free health advice—medical, nutritional, training, fitness questions answered
- Referrals—over 5000 sports medicine health care professionals are on call
- Running shoe database to help you choose the best shoes for your exercise needs.

A catalogue that includes booklets on exercise programs, injury prevention, exercise safety, training, and stretching is also available.

United States Water Fitness Association, Inc.
P.O. Box 3279
Boynton Beach, FL 33424
407-732-9908

Contact: John R. Spannuth, Executive Director

▌ Background

Although crucial to good health and trendy on TV, exercise is a habit of few Americans. Reasons abound; most are excuses. However, many people feel uncomfortable when exercising and still more may be unable to exercise.

Many of the advantages of exercising in gymnasiums and with home equipment can be obtained by exercising in water. Furthermore, water offers the advantage of cushioning the body against injuries, and enabling the elderly and infirmed to exercise regularly.

The United States Water Fitness Association (USWFA), Inc. is a professional, educational, and certifying organization of water fitness instructors who help people exercise in water.

What's Offered

While primarily a professional and educational organization, the USWFA will answer all your questions about water exercising and fitness and will help you find a program or individual instructor in your area.

Additional information about water fitness may be obtained from the Association's publications and videos.

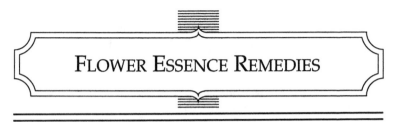

FLOWER ESSENCE REMEDIES

Ellon Bach USA
644 Merrick Road
Lynbrook, NY 11563-2332
800-433-7523

▌ Background

There is no longer any doubt about it. Modern research has confirmed what many alternative healers have known and what many people have intuitively felt: negative emotions and stress can make you sick. They trigger biochemical reactions that weaken the immune system and increase susceptibility to disease and infection.

In the 1920s and 1930s, Dr. Edward Bach developed a theory that certain emotions rendered his patients ill. From this clinical work he developed a series of 38 remedies derived from plants that helped his patients control their feelings of acute stress. They are known throughout the world as the Bach flower remedies.

Ellon Bach USA is a for-profit company selling Bach flower remedies. It is the only authorized distributor of Bach flower remedies.

▌ What's Offered

Ellon Bach's extensive catalogue and questionnaires contain every one of the Bach remedies and information on using them for yourself.

If you believe that you might benefit from this therapy or are just curious about it, this company is an excellent source to start with. A dozen or so books on the remedies and case histories are also offered for sale.

Flower Essence Services
P.O. Box 1769
Nevada City, CA 95959
916-265-0258
916-265-6467 (fax)

▌Background

Other scientists, aside from Dr. Edward Bach, have investigated the health benefits of flower essences. Theories of the potency of flowers date from the writings of Paracelsus in the Middle Ages to Rudolph Steiner in this century. It is only recently that the science of aromatherapy is being seriously investigated in the United States.

Flower Essence Services (FES) conducts field and clinical research in flower essences and has discovered dozens of new ones.

▌What's Offered

FES's extensive series of catalogues contain all the Bach flower remedies, new flower essences used for healing discovered by other researchers, essential plant oils, and a wide variety of publications in the field. They also supply the basic ingredients of many flower essences to allow you to make your own blends.

If you have an interest in flower essences or believe you might benefit from them, this company is an excellent starting point.

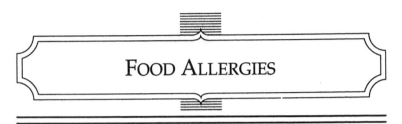

FOOD ALLERGIES

Allergy Alert
P.O. Box 31065
Seattle, WA 98103
206-547-1814

▌ Background

Food: Not the foods that are regarded as unhealthy—fats, sugars, red meat. Not even the artificial additives that are recognized to make at least some people sick. But good food, pure, pesticide-free food, may be some people's worst enemy.

Food sensitivities and intolerances are more common among people who regard themselves as basically healthy than might be imagined. They are common even among people who test negatively when they go to an orthodox allergist.

Allergy Alert is an eight-page, self-help, bimonthly ($18) newsletter written by nutritionist-author, Sally J. Rockwell.

▌ What's Offered

Allergy Alert's breezy style belies the helpful information within. Each issue includes latest research findings on food allergies and sensitivities, cooking tricks to help you avoid certain foods, recipes, and helpful hints presented in little snippets of an easy-to-follow paragraph or two.

Several books of recipes for common food allergy, candidiasis, and hypoglycemic sufferers; a miniseries of food guides on food elimination; starting a food symptom diary; allergy-free baking; and information on rotational diets is also available.

American Celiac Society
58 Musano Court
West Orange, NJ 07052
201-325-8837
215-536-4531

Contact: Annette Bentley, Director and News Editor

▌ Background

Many persons are adversely affected when they eat certain foods; wheat and milk are just two common examples.

The American Celiac Society (ACS) is a grass-roots, self-help organization of people suffering from celiac sprue disease, dermatitus herpetiformis, lactose intolerance, and Crohn's disease.

▌ What's Offered

A yearly ($25) contribution gets you the Society's four-page, quarterly newsletter. The newsletter, written by celiac sufferers, concerns itself with:

- News of members—problems, tips, suggestions
- Food labels—how to avoid what you're allergic to
- Other ailments and symptoms brought on by eating the wrong foods
- Medical breakthroughs in testing and treating these ailments
- Food allergy conference and seminar proceedings.

ACS also regularly reviews and reports on:

- Cookbooks that have recipes its members may eat with no adverse side effects
- Names and addresses of specialty food suppliers
- Legislative lobbying for better food labeling laws.

Gluten Intolerance Group of North America
P.O. Box 23053
Seattle, WA 98102-0353
206-325-6980

Contact: Elaine I. Hartstook, Ph.D.

▌ Background

The one in 2500 persons suffering from celiac sprue, also called gluten sensitivity eneropathy, has inherited an intolerance for gladin-containing proteins found in wheat, rye, barley, and oats. To avoid the symptoms of anemia, chronic fatigue syndrome, muscle cramps, bloating, weight loss, diarrhea, and growth problems in children, people suffering from this allergy must follow a gluten-free diet for life to avoid damage to the lining of their intestines.

The Gluten Intolerance Group (GIG) of North America funds research, reports on the symptoms associated with gluten intolerance, updates gluten-free recipes, reports on foods to avoid, and provides information on forming local support groups.

▌ What's Offered

A $20 membership in GIG includes a subscription to the *GIG Quarterly* containing many useful food tips, recipes, and articles on celiac sprue.

Literature on each of the food-related conditions, all the back issues of the quarterly, several recipe books, and videos are also available.

Mastering Food Allergies
MAST Enterprises, Inc.
2615 North Fourth Street
Suite 616
Coeur d'Alene, ID 83814
208-772-8213

▌ Background

Many persons suffer from one or more food allergies. The most common food allergens are wheat, milk, and corn. *Mastering Food Allergies*, a six-page newsletter published 10 times a year ($20), is aimed at helping allergics to eat better.

▌ What's Offered

The newsletter concentrates on original recipes that are free of common allergens, food preparation tips, medical and health news, physician interviews, information about new food sources, and a regular readers' column. Back issues have covered the following topics and recipes for allergy sufferers:

- Breakfast puddings
- Allergy symptom avoidance in children
- Rotation diet
- Candida and cooking
- Chronic fatigue syndrome
- Biodetoxification
- Asthma
- Homemade baby foods.

MAST also publishes and distributes several cookbooks that have recipes using a single food or recipes that may be used by people suffering from a specific allergen. Topics include:

- Yeast-free cooking

- Baking and cooking with amaranth
- Cooking without common grains.

Further Resources

    see all resources under ORTHOMOLECULAR NUTRITION AND THERAPY

Allergy Information Association

American Academy of Environmental Medicine

Feingold Association of the United States

Practical Allergy Research Foundation

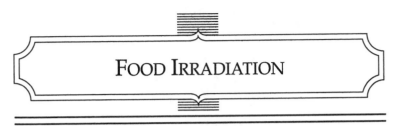

FOOD IRRADIATION

Consumers United for Food Safety
P.O. Box 22928
Seattle, WA 98122
206-747-2659

Contact: Connie Wheeler, Managing Director

▌ Background

Irradiation of food involves the exposure of certain foods to low levels of radioactive materials. Its purpose is to kill microorganisms, insects, and bacteria and to slow down the ripening process.

Opponents believe that nutrients are destroyed when food is irradiated and new, potentially harmful byproducts are created.

At present, irradiation at low levels is approved by the FDA for wheat and wheat flour, potatoes, spices, pork, whole fruits, and vegetables. Only spices are irradiated in larger doses. U.S. law, at the present time, does not require irradiated foods to be labeled as such.

Consumers United for Food Safety (CUFFS) provides information on the dangers of food irradiation and acts as advocates to stop the practice.

▌ What's Offered

A $15 membership to CUFFS entitles you to a four-page, monthly newsletter, *The Food Activist*. Its short articles cover not only the scientific basis for the Society's opposition to food irradiation but the political opposition to the practice. You will also find articles on the use of hormones and other biological agents in food. Recent article topics have included:

■ Dairy farmer—financial impact
■ Milk—use of bovine growth hormone (BGH)
■ Irradiatated food in Florida.

An extensive information packet is available that makes clear their position and shows consumers how to join together in opposition to food irradiation.

Health and Energy Institute
P.O. Box 5357
Tacoma Park, MD 20912
301-585-5541

■ Background

The concern of the Health and Energy Institute's (HEI) is stopping food irradiation. Irradiation is a process of exposing food to low levels of radioactive materials for the purpose of killing microorganisms, insects, and bacteria and slowing the ripening process.

HEI disputes the safety of food irradiation and claims that nutrients are destroyed and new, potentially harmful byproducts are created when food is irradiated. Although approved by the FDA for wheat and wheat flour, potatoes, spices, pork, whole fruits, and vegetables only, spices are irradiated in large amounts. At present, U.S. law does not require irradiated foods to be labeled as such.

▌ What's Offered

Believing that all sources of ionizing radiation that can be avoided should be, the Institute publishes pamphlets and booklets directed at the lay public, conducts its own scientific research, provides reports and studies of other concerned groups, organizes seminars and workshops, and testifies before legislative bodies.

Publication and brochure topics include:

- ▌ Women's exposure to radiation
- ▌ Radiation hazards on the job
- ▌ Atomic radiation
- ▌ Food irradiation basics.

HEI also provides information on the risks of exposure to all other sources of ionizing radiation including dental and medical X-rays, and CAT scans.

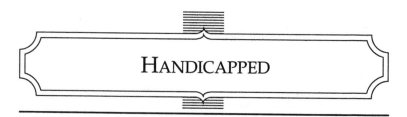

HANDICAPPED

National Handicapped Sports
1145 19th Street, NW
Suite 717
Washington, DC 20036
301-652-7505
301-652-0119 (TDD for hearing impaired)
301-652-0790 (fax)

▌ Background

The motto of National Handicapped Sports (NHS) is "If I Can Do This I Can Do Anything." NHS' stated mission is to make certain that every handicapped individual is able to maximize his or her fitness goals.

▌ What's Offered

A $15 membership in NHS includes a subscription to *Handicapped Sports Report*, a tabloid-sized, quarterly newspaper with stories of handicapped athletes and sporting events.

NHS offers "Fitness for Everyone" courses in strength, flexibility, and aerobic conditioning and several fitness videos for paraplegics, quadraplegics, cerebral palsy victims, and amputees. They also sponsor winter ski programs for the disabled and many youth programs. Associated with many sports associations and with its own local chapters across the country, NHS plans many sport and recreational activities throughout the year.

Society for the Advancement of Travel for the Handicapped
26 Court Street
Brooklyn, NY 11242
718-858-5483
718-596-6310 (fax)

Contact: Mark Shaw

▌ Background

Many handicapped people don't travel. They are embarrassed by their disability or believe that there are no means provided for them to get around comfortably.

The Society for the Advancement of Travel for the Handicapped (SATH) was formed to provide information to the handicapped and disabled who wanted to travel.

▌ What's Offered

A $40 membership to SATH will bring you their eight-page, quarterly *SATH News*. Its short articles highlight what's available to the traveling handicapped or disabled person. Articles cover special programs, scuba, and museum tours; accessibility at airports, hotels, and tourist sites; travel clubs and travel agents serving the handicapped; and special sporting events.

SATH has also prepared a resource directory on the many travel services now available for the handicapped and reviews commercial and government publications that focus on these services.

Further Resources
National Information Center for Children and Youth with Handicaps

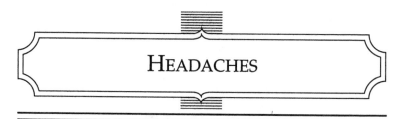

Headaches

American Council For Health Education
875 Kings Highway
West Deptford, NJ 08096
800-255-ACHE

▌ Background

Almost everyone has headaches from time to time. But 50 million Americans suffer from severe headaches on a regular basis. Most do not know whether their headaches are migraine, cluster, or tension-related headaches. Too many do no more than take an over-the-counter preparation and learn to live with the pain.

Yet by even the most orthodox estimates, at least 20% of all headaches are related to diet. Many are the result of environmental factors or stress. No pharmaceutical would do more than temporarily relieve the symptoms, while alternative diagnosis and treatment might make those headaches entirely a thing of the past.

The American Council For Health Education (ACHE) disseminates information to the general public and headache sufferers on all types of headaches and the wide range of approaches that help their sufferers.

▌ What's Offered

A telephone call will get you several brochures on different headache types; how to easily tell if they're related to diet, stress, or the environment; and a sample issue of a free, four-page, monthly newsletter, *ACHE Newsletter*. Regular features include answers to readers' questions. All the articles are short and nontechnical and discuss only the practical aspects of headache relief. Recent article topics from several issues are:

- Nutrasweet^{TM} and migraine
- Medicine misuse
- Headache myths
- Aspirin and migraine prevention
- Tyramine-restricted diets
- Ancient headache treatments.

National Headache Foundation
5252 North Western Avenue
Chicago, IL 60625
800-843-2256
312-878-7725

▌ Background

While just about everyone knows that back pain is the most common health complaint, few people are aware that headaches are the second. Millions of people suffer chronic, often debilitating, headaches.

The National Headache Foundation (NHF) serves both headache sufferers and their families, as well as health care professionals. NHF's three major goals are:

- To serve as a source of information for the two groups
- To promote research into the cause and treatment of various types of headaches
- To educate the general public about the seriousness of headaches.

▌ What's Offered

The NHF's information on headache causes and treatments is free. Be sure to mention the type of headache you are interested in or at least its symptoms when you write and enclose a self-addressed, double-stamped envelope. If you request it, a list of headache specialists for your state will also be included.

If you have a serious interest or are a chronic headache sufferer you may wish to join ($15) the Foundation. Membership entitles you to their quarterly newsletter, several brochures on headaches and their treatment, information on biofeedback and headaches, and much more. The newsletter will keep you up to date on headache research, new theories on headache causes, and clinical reports on the latest treatments.

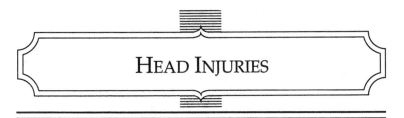

HEAD INJURIES

National Head Injury Foundation, Inc.
1140 Connecticut Avenue, NW
Suite 812
Washington, DC 20036
202-296-6443
800-444-NHIF (Hotline)
202-296-8850 (fax)

Contact: Patricia Stedman, Resources Coordinator

▌ Background

Head and brain injuries are a growing phenomenon. In spite of increased auto safety—seat belts, child restraints, air bags; and the use of helmets—motorcycle and bicycle—more and more people are sustaining such injuries.

The National Head Injury Foundation (NHIF), Inc. was founded to improve the quality of life for survivors of head injuries and to promote the prevention of head injuries through public education. Its focuses are:

- ▌ State associations of support groups
- ▌ Legal and medical advocacy
- ▌ Educational and research activities
- ▌ Health care professionals council.

▌ What's Offered

Membership in NHIF is $35 or extended as a courtesy to those who have sustained a brain injury or their family members and are unable to pay. NHIF provides the following services for its members:

- Answer questions about head injuries and their consequences
- Provide detailed information about specific aspects of head injury
- Referrals to health care professionals
- Link people to a nationwide network of patients and their families.

NHIF also has a 100-page-plus catalogue of written material, audio tapes, and videos on head injuries. The material ranges from booklets addressed to patients to treatment modalities addressed to clinicians. The material covers general information, prevention, family issues, rehabilitation, treatment, related neurological disorders, pediatrics, coping, and legal matters.

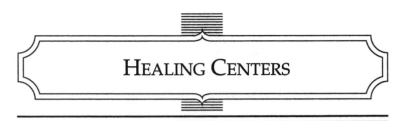

HEALING CENTERS

Association of Holistic Healing Centers
2100 Mediterranean Avenue
Suite 40
Virginia Beach, VA 23451
804-498-2598

▮ Background

What is clearly and consciously missing from this book are alternative treatment centers and healing clinics. To have included them would have made this book three times its present size and would imply an endorsement (at least implicitly by its inclusion) of their treatments. Instead, I have provided you with information sources from which you can not only get a great deal of self-help information, but from which you may also get information on and referrals to clinics and centers.

However, that may be insufficient at times. Many centers provide services that are so radical that they may not fit into a predefined category. Many centers do not promote themselves beyond their own community. Many are not located in the United States.

For those reasons I have included the Association of Holistic Healing Centers, a professional organization of individuals, groups, and centers involved in healing. Its stated mission is:

- ▮ To educate its members
- ▮ To sponsor conferences, workshops and seminars
- ▮ To create prototype healing centers.

■ What's Offered

Membership ($35) is open to anyone involved or interested in the healing arts and includes a quarterly newsletter and periodic reports on and invitations to international tours, conferences, and workshops.

For health care consumers seeking a referral or further information on the healing arts, a directory of members is available.

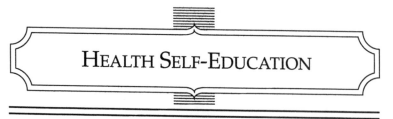

HEALTH SELF-EDUCATION

Aurora Book Companions
P.O. Box 5852
Denver, CO 80217

■ Background

A company selling health books is hardly an alternative health care resource, yet this one is. Simply put, Aurora Book Companions is one of the best places to order a health book when you cannot find it in your library or at your local health food store or book store.

■ What's Offered

Write for Aurora's free color catalogue and within a week it will be delivered to your mailbox. In it you will find thousands and thousands of books on every health topic you can think of (and many that you may never even have heard of). Some of the more popular health topics include:

- Allergies
- Back and spine problems
- Alternative healing
- Childbirth and care
- Cooking
- Dental problems
- Headaches
- Seasonal affective disorders.

Needless to say, I have left out hundreds of topics, each one with more than a dozen books on alternative health and therapies in it. You may return any book you find unsatisfactory, and discounts for many books are common.

Health Resource
209 Katherine Drive
Conway, AR 72032
501-329-5272
501-329-8700 (fax)

Contact: Janice R. Guthrie

▌ Background

It is not difficult to find at least some information on just about any health issue or medical problem. But what if you do not have the time, or you need detailed information, or the subject is an obscure one?

For those seeking customized health and medical information, Health Resource may be of value.

▌ What's Offered

Health Resource provides individualized reports on specific health issues or medical problems. Each report runs between 50 and 150 pages and will provide you with:

- Treatment options—advantages, disadvantages
- Research—new treatments, risks, benefits
- Self-help measures
- Physicians specializing in the disease or condition
- Lists of books and other research material
- Resource organizations and government agencies for follow-up information.

The information is gathered from medical texts and journals, health books and magazines, medical school and university libraries, and computer databases.

=======

Lafayette University
941 South Havana Street
Aurora, CO 80012
303-341-0082
303-341-0084

▌ Background

The general area of health care subjects taught in the Department of Holistic Health and Wellness Studies at Lafayette University includes:

- Chiropathy—a pastoral therapeutic method to help the body rejuvenate itself
- Nutritional science
- Botanical medicine
- Imagery.

▌ What's Offered

Although a Christian-based pastoral college, theologians teach courses in nonhealth subjects and only health care professionals train health care professionals-to-be in subjects such as:

- Counseling
- Hypnotherapy
- Nutrition
- Herbology
- Polarity therapy
- Botanical studies

■ Visual therapy
■ Wellness.

Besides Lafayette University's courses and degree programs, they will be happy to provide you with referrals to health care practitioners and counselors in your area.

Planetree Health Resource
2041 Webster Street
San Francisco, CA 94115
415-923-3680

Contact: Elizabeth U. Schwartz

■ Background

You can be an active participant in your health or you may passively accept the advice and treatment of others. There are no other choices.
Planetree Health Resource seeks to provide consumers of health and medical care with the information they need to become active participants.

■ What's Offered

A $35 yearly membership allows you to access all Planetree's facilities and personnel. For the nonresident of San Francisco these include access to their library and the purchase of specially prepared material.
You may borrow from their library of standard medical texts, health care books, alternative health care material, medical journals, health newsletters, audio tapes, and videos.
In-depth health care packets on various illnesses that include recent articles, orthodox and complementary therapy options, a computerized bibliography, reprints from medical texts and con-

sumer health periodicals, and a list of national and local health and support organizations are also available for purchase.

Tree Farm Communications
23703 NE Fourth Street
Redmond, WA 98053
206-868-0464
206-868-8652 (fax)

Contact: Jay Johnson

■ Background

Many professional organizations hold conferences, seminars, and workshops at which new techniques, treatments, and information that could prevent disease are presented. The information at these events often takes decades to become known even in the alternative health care community. It may take 40 years before it becomes a part of the cultural mainstream.

Tree Farm Communications records many of these events and makes them available on audio cassettes.

■ What's Offered

Write or telephone for a catalogue. In it you will find dozens of conference proceedings. Several topics discussed at recent health food conferences are:

- Medicinal herbs
- Vascular cleansing
- Garlic
- Skin care
- Amino acids
- Pain and stress.

More topics from several naturopathic associations, an alternative treatment symposium, and a World Congress on Natural Medicine held in Malaga, Spain, included:

- Food enzyme therapy
- Botanical medicine
- Nutrition and prevention
- Psoriasis
- Parkinson's disease
- Diabetes mellitus
- AIDS
- Women's health forum
- Light-wave acupuncture
- Autism
- Iris diagnosis
- Environmental pollution
- Bioresonance.

Tree Farm's audios are $9 per tape, with a discount for an entire conference. There are also many individual lectures from some of the foremost alternative health care pioneers and several complete courses in herbology.

World Research Foundation
15300 Ventura Boulevard
Suite 405
Sherman Oaks, CA 91403
818-907-5483
818-907-6044 (fax)

Background

Wouldn't it be nice to be able to search the world's literature to find alternative health care and prevention information that's often unavailable in the Unted States?

Gathering and making available information on health and the environment from around the world is the major purpose of the World Research Foundation.

▐ What's Offered

The information available to the public falls under three broad categories:

- Listings and details of various alternative health care and preventive techniques discovered
- The effects of various drugs and their ingredients
- Lectures, seminars, publictions, audio tapes, and videos on new alternative techniques.

Library searches are from the Foundation's collection of more than 5000 journals from 100 countries and 100,000 books. Almost all contain complementary, nontraditional, alternative, and natural therapies or preventive regimens.

Computer searches access more than 500 databases that normally contain the tradiitonal pharmaceutical and surgical treatments that your medical doctor should know about before using it on you, but often does not.

A minimum donation entitles you to receive the Foundation's quarterly *World Research Journal* that contains information about its upcoming seminars, new publications, and new medical and health techniques. Recent issues have discussed:

- Acupuncture
- Color, sound, and music therapies
- Magnetic healing
- Visualization.

Further Resources
American Institute of Biomedical Climatology
Lloyd Library and Museum
MEDLARS
NAPRALERT

HEARING PROBLEMS

Self Help for Hard of Hearing People, Inc.
7800 Wisconsin Avenue
Bethesda, MD 20814
301-657-2248

▌ Background

Hearing loss affects many people as they grow older. What is not as well known is the rising problem of hearing loss among children and young adults.

Self Help for Hard of Hearing People (Shhh), Inc. was founded to counteract the ignorance most people have about hearing loss and to act as an information resource to those who are sufferers. Focusing on self-help, its purposes are:

- To create public awareness about hearing loss
- To implement special programs for the hearing impaired
- To publish practical information on hearing loss and the help that is available
- To represent the hard of hearing to the health care community
- To improve communications access in theaters, telephones, and TV.

▌ What's Offered

A $15 membership to Shhh includes the bimonthly: *Shhh Journal*. Its article topics have included:

- Hearing impairment in the workplace
- Hearing aids—T-switch, audio induction loops

- Psychological stress and hearing loss
- Genetics and hearing impairment
- Tinnitus
- Hard-of-hearing children
- Noise—health problems
- Sensorineural hearing loss—rehabilitation
- Closed-captioned decoders.

Shhh publishes many short technical articles on hearing loss and listening-aid devices that are available. There are several hundred local individual chapters throughout the country offering self-help, support, and local newsletters.

Referrals to health care practitioners and advice about hearing aids or any other problems relating to hearing loss are answered on an individual basis.

Further Resources
American Speech-Language Hearing Association

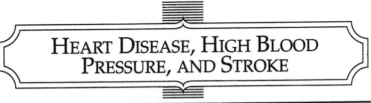

HEART DISEASE, HIGH BLOOD PRESSURE, AND STROKE

Cardiac Alert
Phillips Publishing, Inc.
7811 Montrose Road
P.O. Box 61350
Potomac, MD 20897-5405
800-777-5005

▌ Background

The leading cause of death in the United States—35.3% of deaths every year—is heart disease. Many of those deaths can be prevented, or at least postponed for a time, with lifestyle changes.

The monthly ($39) *Cardiac Alert* has one purpose: to provide you with information on how you can prevent a heart attack through positive lifestyle changes.

▌ What's Offered

Although not exclusively a source for alternative health care information, far more than the all too common prescriptions of surgery and pharmaceuticals are presented each month.

It will take you about half an hour to go through this lively, eclectic newsletter. It has no technical terms or jargon, no lengthy explanations, just short and pithy articles on the latest research findings, prevention, recovery, and how you can implement each one in your life. Some samples of recent article topics are:

- ▪ Cutting medicine costs—with or without insurance
- ▪ Blood pressure testing—which tests count

- Dietary considerations for the heart
- HDL and LDL cholesterol—getting the right balance
- Nutrition and the heart—what to do
- Foods that reverse heart disease
- Exercising—when and how much
- Brain angina—what is it and how to prevent it
- Elective surgery after a heart attack.

Heart Disease Research Foundation
50 Court Street
Brooklyn, NY 11201
718-649-6210

▌ Background

While heart disease is still a major killer in America, medical orthodoxy has contributed far less than changes in lifestyle to its prevention and cure. Lowering your blood pressure, cholesterol, and stress, quitting cigarette smoking, following a rational diet, exercising, and having proper nutrient supplementation will go farther in preventing a heart attack, speeding its recovery, and extending the lives of its victims than any surgical procedure or drug.

The Heart Disease Research Foundation (HDRF) aims its heart research at early diagnosis, prevention, and treatment. The alternative methods of treatment that have been investigated include the effects of acupuncture and electrotherapy on blood chemistry and the cardiovascular system.

▌ What's Offered

There are no costs associated with the information you will get from the HDRF. The only price is the effort you exert to understand it. The information is written by doctors for doctors and research scientists. Nevertheless, if you make the effort it will prove worth your while. Subjects include:

■ Prevention of cardiovascular diseases
■ Fat in the diet and the development of atherosclerosis
■ Dietary factors other than fat on the cardiovascular system
■ Nutrition, diet, and cholesterol in cardiovascular disease.

HOPE Heart Institute
350 East Michigan Avenue
Suite 301
Kalamazoo, MI 49007-3857
616-343-0770

■ Background

Associated with a health research institute, HOPE Heart Institute publishes several books and a newsletter on health-related topics for the general public.

■ What's Offered

Its monthly ($19.80) newsletter, *The HOPE Health Letter*, has short, lively, easy-to-follow articles. The primary purpose of the material is to convey preventive information on diet, nutrition, and heart disease in easy-to-understand language and a pleasant format. It's definitely for the lay reader. Recent issues have discussed the following topics:

■ HDL and LDL cholesterol levels
■ Keeping your own medical records
■ Fitness—diet and exercise

- Risks of heart disease—performing a self-test
- Weight loss
- Flus and colds—what works and what doesn't.

A catalogue of other health materials and books, all written for the lay individual, is also available.

Linus Pauling Institute of Science and Medicine
400 Page Mill Road
Palo Alto, CA 94306-2025
415-327-4064
415-327-8564 (fax)

Contact: Richard Hicks, Executive Vice President

■ Background

More people in the United States visit their doctor for high blood pressure, known as hypertension, than for any other reason. Consequently, more prescriptions are written for high blood pressure than any other ailment. Estimates are that 60%—that's more than 30%—of the adult population suffer from high blood pressure.

Associated with hypertension is heart disease, especially the heart attack or stroke. Of the 1.5 million yearly heart attacks, fewer than 350,000 victims survive.

■ What's Offered

Dr. Mathias Rath and Dr. Linus Pauling, doing research under the auspices of the Institute, have come up with some remarkable results regarding cardiovascular disease and its relation to Vitamin C.

In a series of articles published in the *Proceedings of the National Academy of Science* (vol. 87, August 1990, pp. 6204-6207, Chemistry; and vol. 87, December 1990, pp. 9388-9390, Biochemistry) and *The Journal of Orthomolecular Medicine* (vol. 6, nos. 3 and 4, pp. 125–133, 139–143), they have demonstrated that a deficiency of ascorbate (vitamin C) leads to increasing deposits of a special type of lipoprotein—lipoprotein a—on blood vessel walls. The presence of lipoprotein a is directly related to the incidence of cardiovascular disease in both humans and other mammals that do not themselves manufacture their required ascorbate.

The conclusions are telling. An increase of vitamin C to what are now considered megadoses by establishment medicine may prevent many, if not most, forms of cardiovascular disease. Megadoses of vitamin C may also help reverse long-term damage to blood vessels, even in those who have already had a heart attack. Both these conclusions prove true even in those with a genetic pre-disposition toward cardiovascular illness.

Stroke Foundation, Inc.
898 Park Avenue
New York, NY 10021
212-734-3461

▌ Background

Four hundred thousand Americans suffer a stroke every year. Close to two-thirds of those surviving may be handicapped or disabled. While medical research has done much to increase the survival rate of stroke victims, changes in lifestyle can do more to prevent it than anything else yet available from medical science.

The Stroke Foundation, Inc. provides funds for research grants, stroke training for physicians, and education programs for stroke prevention. It is not an alternative health care organization, but one that stresses prevention.

▌ What's Offered

Drop them a letter and you will receive a small information packet containing a booklet on stroke and excerpts from medical publications that tell of several lifestyle changes that can decrease your chances of suffering a stroke.

Further Resources
    see all resources under ALTERNATIVE HEALING
    see all resources under CHELATION THERAPY
    see all resources under FITNESS
    see all resources under LIFESTYLE
    see all resources under NUTRITION AND DIET
    see all resources under ORTHOMOLECULAR NUTRITION AND
        THERAPY
    see all resources under STRESS REDUCTION
    Cancer Control Society

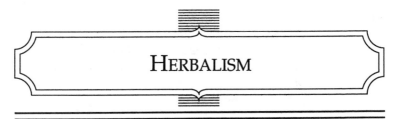

HERBALISM

American Botanical Council
P.O. Box 201660
Austin, TX 78720-1660
512-331-8868
512-331-924 (fax)

▌ Background

The American Botanical Council (ABC) is a research and educational organization dedicated to providing reliable research data on herbs as medicines, foods, and cosmetics. Its objectives are:

- ▌ To support research on herbal folk remedies, teas, and other herb-based products
- ▌ To publish accurate research findings from around the world
- ▌ To act as a forum between herbalists, physicians, scientists, and interested individuals
- ▌ To be a reliable source of information on medicinal plants.

▌ What's Offered

ABCs premier publication (published in association with the Herb Research Foundation) is its quarterly ($30) *HerbalGram*. This lavishly illustrated journal will keep you fascinated for hours. Regular columns include readers' letters, book reviews, and a calendar of coming events. Recent issues have included extensive information on:

- ▌ Hawthorn berries as a heart tonic
- ▌ Sesame flower treatment for warts

- Ephedra—chemical constituents and therapeutic benefits
- Herbal oral contraceptives
- Report on the European Congress on Phytotherapy
- Psychotropic botanicals.

Back issues and reprints of major articles are available.

American Herb Association
P.O. Box 353
Rescue, CA 95672
916-626-5046
916-492-0955 (fax)

▌ Background

The American Herb Association (AHA) promotes herbal education and seeks to increase the use of herbs and herbal products by both laypersons and professionals in healing while conducting independent research in the medicinal uses of herbs and herbal products.

▌ What's Offered

A $20 yearly membership in the AHA will entitle you to a subscription to the *American Herb Quarterly Newsletter*. In it you will find short, lively, and well-researched articles on topics such as:

- Up-to-date research on herbal health
- Herb gardening
- New herbal products
- Book reviews
- Consumer reports.

The Association also publishes several herbal source directories to help you find seeds and plants and herbal items and products. They will be happy to send you a sample issue of their newsletter for $4.

Herb Research Foundation
1007 Pearl Street
Suite 200
Boulder, CO 80302
303-449-2265

Contact: Carolyn Colwill

▌ Background

The oldest medicines were made from the plant kingdom—botanicals. Even today, with all that modern biochemistry and genetic engineering can do, more than 40% of all pharmaceuticals in the United States come from plants.

The Herb Research Foundation is the foremost herb research organization in the country. It conducts independent research on uses of herbs and their safety and disseminates reliable, scientific information on botanical medicines to professionals and the general public.

▌ What's Offered

Their $25 membership entitles you to a subscription to the 52-page, color quarterly, *HerbalGram* (published in association with the American Botanical Council).

Other services include computerized botanical literature searching, several pamphlets and abstract files on individual herbs.

Lloyd Library and Museum
917 Plum Street
Cincinnati, OH 45202
513-721-3707

▌ Background

The oldest known form of medicines is herbals. Throughout the history of the world much has been written on the health and restorative benefit of botanical preparations.

The Lloyd Library and Museum, founded by John, Curtis, and Nelson Lloyd, manufacturing pharmacists, houses one of the world's largest and most unique collections of books and periodicals dating back to 1493 on herbals, eclectic medicine, and pharmacognosy.

The information at the Lloyd Library is so extensive and unique that the U.S. National Library of Medicine often recommends its own patrons to go there for information that cannot be obtained elsewhere.

▌ What's Offered

Anyone may use the library. If any information cannot be found in the library's collection, they will contact other sources to get you an answer. The Lloyd Library prides itself on the fact that "no patron is ever turned away empty."

If you cannot visit its facilities, write to them and they will be happy to get you an answer to any questions on herbal preparations and botanical medicine and send it back to you by letter, photocopy, or microfilm.

Medical Herbalism
P.O. Box 33080
Portland, OR 97233

Background

Medical Herbalism, a 12-page newsletter published six times a year
($18) focuses on the use of herbs as medicines. Although aimed at
the professional herbalist, he or she is as likely to be a lay practitioner, as a medical professional.

What's Offered

Medical Herbalism does not discuss theory. Instead, its concern is
the practical application of herbalism. It is eclectic in approach: not
overly devoted to any one school of thought or practice. Articles
are usually no more than a page or two long and often give
formulations and case histories. Examples of topics covered in
recent issues include:

- Comfrey—uses and preparations
- Whole herbs and active ingredients
- Rheumatoid arthritis—herbal treatments
- Hydrotherapy
- Ginkgo biloba—chemical constituents
- Hypericum and AIDS
- CAGE test for alcoholism.

Phyto-Pharmica Review
Vital Communications, Inc.
12819 Southeast 38th Street
Suite 159
Bellevue, WA 98006
206-286-5966

Contact: Michael T. Murray, N.D.

■ Background

Phyto-Pharmica Review is a monthly newslettter devoted to a single topic—botanical medicine.

■ What's Offered

Written by a naturopathic physician, Dr. Michael T. Murray, this is a straightforward, nonjargon, scientific journal. The articles are no more than a page or two long, thoroughly researched, well documented, and with many references and citations. Most often it is addressed to other professional clinicians, but the interested individual will still get much valuable information. Several recent issues have discussed:

- ■ Sources of dietary fiber
- ■ Coleus forskohli—an ayruvedic medicine
- ■ Botanical menopause treatments.

By the way, excerpts from many issues come as inserts in the *Townsend Letter for Doctors.*

Therapeutic Herbalism
9304 Springhill School Road
Sebastopol, CA 95472

▌ Background

Information on herbalism abounds: books, specialized periodicals, and general health magazines. But what do you do if you want more but do not want to make a career of it?

Therapeutic Herbalism is a home-study correspondence course on the foundations of modern herbal therapeutics and European phytotherapy.

▌ What's Offered

The course's preparer, David Hoffman, is a member of Great Britain's National Institute of Medical Herbalism and past president of the American Herbalist Guild. He is not only an herbalist and teacher but the author of six books on herbalism for both the general public and standard texts for the profession.

The course is designed to provide a foundation for anyone interested in self-help, herbal health care and provides a means for maintenance and disease prevention. But this is not a course that will make you a professional herbalist, nor will it replace the benefits of seeking the advice of a professional at all times.

Its curriculum falls into six broad areas:

- ▌ Therapeutic herbalism—information sources and approaches
- ▌ Herbal actions—physiological mechanisms, primary and secondary actions, therapeutic implications
- ▌ Body systems—tonic herbs health maintenance and disease prevention

- Materia medica of 200 plants—actions, indications, contrain-
  dications, dosage
- Phytopharmacology
- Medicine making.

Further Resources
  see all resources under FLOWER ESSENCE REMEDIES
    NAPRALERT

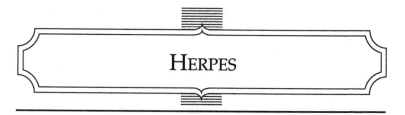

HERPES

American Social Health Association
Herpes Resource Center
P.O. Box 13827
Research Triangle Park, NC 27709
919-361-8422
919-361-2120 (Herpes hotline)

▌ Background

The most common chronic condition is a sexually transmitted disease (STD): herpes. It is estimated that 31 million adults have genital herpes and 100 million have oral herpes.

The stated mission of the American Social Health Association (ASHA) Herpes Resource Center (HRC) is:

- To create and distribute educational material on herpes
- To expand medical and social support
- To advocate for a national policy toward all STDs including herpes
- To fund research.

▌ What's Offered

ASHA by no means provides alternative health care information about herpes, but they do provide information, some of which includes nonconventional treatments.

The Center provides a number of free pamphlets and makes available several audio tapes and videos. A $25 membership fee will include a subscription to the HRC's quarterly, *The Helper*. Articles are prepared by recognized experts, contain up-to-date herpes information and research findings, and are directed toward the general public. Some topics covered from recent issues are:

- Herpes and pregnancy
- DMSO—topical additive
- BHT—treatment
- Natural immunomodulators
- Effect of nutrients—water-soluble vitamins
- Vitamin C ascorbate.

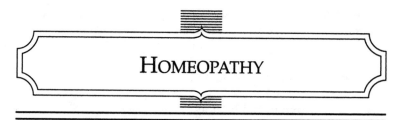

HOMEOPATHY

Biological Therapy
Menaco
P.O. Box 11280
Albuquerque, NM 87192

▌ Background

Biological Therapy, a quarterly ($10) scientific journal, published
under the auspices of a company manufacturing and selling homeopathic preparations to professionals (Biological Homeopathic
Industries), calls itself the "Journal of Natural Medicine."

▌ What's Offered

Pick up any issue and you are likely to find six to eight articles.
Most are clinical reports from physicians and homeopaths; the rest
are studies of the effectiveness of homeopathic medicines. Some
articles are reprinted from foreign medical journals. All are thoroughly researched, have extensive references, and are written primarily for the professional clinician.

If you are interested in homeopathy and want to learn more
about which medicines may prove effective for you, then this
journal may be of interest. But be forewarned, the reading is not
easy. Some recent article topics are:

- ▌ Achilles tendonitus
- ▌ Digestive disorders and homeopathic preparations
- ▌ Tonsillitis
- ▌ Homotoxicology theory

- Chronic disorder therapy
- Influenza in young chilldren.

Homeopathic Academy of Naturopathic Physicians
14653 Graves Road
Mulino, OR 97042
503-829-7326
503-829-7326 (fax)

▌Background

As with most things that survive (and flourish), homeopathy also has many different schools of thought and professional practice.

The Homeopathic Academy of Naturopathic Physicians (HANP) is a professional organization of Naturopaths (N.D.s) who use classical homeopathy as one of their treatment modalities.

The HANP's purpose is:

- To encourage and to improve the homeopathic curriculum at naturopathic colleges
- To set educational and professional standards for practice and certification
- To provide continuing professional education and training.

▌What's Offered

As with almost all professional organizations, HANP publishes a journal, *Simillimum*. This quarterly's ($40) articles are primarily devoted to clinical studies and reports of successful uses of classical homeopathic medicines for treatment of both common ailments and degenerative diseases. Other article topics relate to professional practices and news of upcoming events. Topics on clinical cases for a recent issue are:

- Strep throat
- Acute dizziness
- Lupus and arthritis
- Measles.

Of more concern to health care consumers is that HANP also maintains a referral list of naturopaths who use classical homeopathy in their practice and will be happy to make a referral to one in your area if you write or telephone.

Homeopathic Educational Services
2124 Kittredge Street
Berkeley, CA 94704
415-649-0294
415-649-1955 (fax)

▌ Background

Homeopathy is a natural pharmaceutical science utilizing very small doses of individually prescribed substances that stimulate the immune system to cure a malady.

Homeopathic Educational Services (HES) provides general information on homeopathy in the form of books, audio tapes, medicines, software, and kits.

▌ What's Offered

If you already have an interest in homeopathy or would just like to find out about it, any one of the hundreds of books, courses, and audios offered by this mail-order firm will satisfy you. HES has materials for beginners and experts and for the layperson and the physician, on the philosophical and the practical level and on children's preparations and veterinary homeopathy.

You may also buy already prepared homeopathic medicines for minor ailments such as acne, sore throats, hay fever, and headache, as well as homeopathic medicine kits, audio tapes, software, and so forth.

International Foundation for Homeopathy

2366 Eastlake Avenue East
Suite 301
Seattle, WA 98102
206-324-8230

▌ Background

The International Foundation for Homeopathy (IFH) promotes homeopathic science through professional education; it trains health care practitioners in homeopathy, conducts seminars for the interested individual, and presents professional seminars, conferences and workshops to encourge public awareness of classical homeopathy.

▌ What's Offered

A $25 membership in the IFH includes a first-aid chart, a national directory of classical homeopaths, and a subscription to *Resonance*, a bimonthly, 12-page magazine of articles describing homeopathic remedies through case studies.

Serving as a clearinghouse for information, the Foundation will be happy to answer your questions on homeopathy and provide you with a referral to a classical homeopath in your area.

National Center for Homeopathy
1500 Massachusetts Avenue, NW
Suite 42
Washington, DC 20005
202-223-6182

▌ Background

Homeopathy is based upon three principles:

▌ Like cures like—the unique symptoms of the ailment are matched by the remedy

▌ Single remedy—Only a single medicine is given at any one time

▌ Minimum dose—only the smallest possible dose is given to minimize possible adverse side effects.

Homeopathic practitioners diagnose illnesses and prescribe homeopathic medicines. These medicines, for both acute and chronic conditions manufactured from natural sources and to precise potencies, are used to stimulate self-healing.

The National Center for Homeopathy (NCH), the governing body of many professional homeopaths, views part of its mission as preserving medical freedom of choice. The other half is to provide continuing homeopathic education for both the professional practitioner and the interested individual.

▌ What's Offered

A $35 membership includes a subscription to the NCH's monthly 24-page newsletter, *Homeopathy Today*. It contains newsy articles on homeopathic education: conferences, seminars, and workshops; clinical notes; and legislative matters.

Many books on practical homeopathy for the layperson along with several homeopathic kits are also available.

The Center will also provide you with a "Directory of Homeopathic Practitioners," from which you can find a professional in your area.

HOSPICE

Children's Hospice, International
1101 King Street
Suite 131
Alexandria, VA 22314
703-684-0330
800-2-4-CHILD (hotline)

▌ Background

We all know that everyone who was ever born will someday die.
But perhaps the hardest thing to accept is the death of a child,
someone who has never really tasted life. It's all the harder when
that child dies slowly from a disease that slowly steals his or her
life.

The Children's Hospice, International (CHI) provides a support system for health care professionals and the families of termi-
nally ill children.

▌ What's Offered

Membership in CHI ($35) is open to everyone and includes a
quarterly newsletter and product discounts. But no one need join
to take advantage of CHI's services. Information in the form of
audio tapes and books not only discusses hospice but parental
bereavement, trauma, and childhood death.

You may also call their hotline for answers to any questions
about children and dying, parental bereavement, and how you
may go about finding a children's hospice if you need one.

National Hospice Organization
1901 North Moore Street
Suite 901
Arlington, VA 22209
800-658-8898 (hotline)
703-243-5900

▮ Background

Many people are more afraid of dying than of death. They especially fear dying from a terminal illness and the associated pain,
helplessness, fear, loneliness, and the feeling that the hospital or
nursing home is merely waiting until someone else can use the bed.

An alternative to dying alone in a hospital or nursing home
is a hospice. The National Hospice Organization (NHO) is an
organization of hospice providers that seeks to make the general
public more aware of this option and integrate hospices into the
health care system.

▮ What's Offered

NHO will help you decide if a hospice is a viable alternative by
providing you with information about what you can expect from
a hospice. They will help you find out if there's a hospice near you
and tell you of the benefits of hospice care versus hospital care.

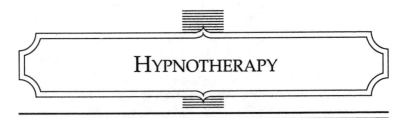

HYPNOTHERAPY

Academy of Scientific Hypnotherapy
P.O. Box 12041
San Diego, CA 92112
619-427-6225

Contact: Dr. William E. Kemery

▌ Background

Hypnosis is an intense form of relaxation. More than that alone, hypnosis is an altered conscious mental state in which the mind can focus on particular details and banish extraneous thoughts. It is characterized by a sense of relaxation and high suggestibility.

Very much a part of alternative medicine, hypnosis has had success in treating anxiety, phobias, obesity, high blood pressure, depression, neuroses, abnormal heart rhythms, asthma, headaches, seizures, arthritis, and surgery pain.

The Academy of Scientific Hypnotherapy (ASH) acts as a clearinghouse, a common ground where professional hypnotherapists and people seeking their help can come together.

▌ What's Offered

More than anything else, ASH acts as a referral service. Write or telephone, being sure to state what you want a hypnotherapist for, and a referral to a specialist in your area will be sent back to you.

Hypnotherapy in Review, the Academy's major publication, has reported the benefits of hypnosis in:

- Reduced bleeding in hemophiliacs
- Birthing
- Criminal cases.

American Academy of Medical Hypnoanalysts
710 East Ogden Avenue
Suite 208
Naperville, IL 60563
800-34-HYPNO

Background

One way of helping people with psychological problems is through hypnosis. It is often used as a tool to help people relax or allow them to regress back to childhood to relive their experiences.

However, hypnosis may also be used as the therapeutic agency itself. The purpose of the American Academy of Medical Hypnoanalysts is to train professional psychotherapists in the use of hypnosis as a medical procedure.

What's Offered

Membership in the American Academy of Medical Hypnoanalysts (AAMH) is only available to professionals who also receive the Academy's quarterly, *Medical Hypnoanalysis Journal.*

A national referral service is available. The AAMH will help you find psychotherapists who use hypnosis in your area.

American Guild of Hypnotherapists
4532 West Napoleon Avenue
Metarie, LA 70001
504-455-5708

Contact: Dr. Grace Lee

∎ Background

Hypnosis, aside from its show business image, is used throughout
the world as a therapeutic means of altering behavior and changing
habits.

The American Guild of Hypnotherapists is a professional
accreditation organization that conducts educational seminars and
workshops and promotes standards of treatment.

∎ What's Offered

The Guild's official publication, the quarterly *Journal of Hypnotherapy*, serves as a continuing educational medium in the practice of
hypnotherapy as a therapy.

Referrals to a professional hypnotist or hypnotherapist in
your area are available by telephone or letter.

American Society of Clinical Hypnosis
2200 East Devon
Suite 291
Des Plaines, IL 60018
708-297-3317
708-297-7309 (fax)

Contact: William F. Hoffman, Jr., Executive Vice President

▌ Background

Many health care professionals use hypnosis in their clinical practice. Aside from the obvious psychological benefits to those professionals practicing psychotherapy, dentists and doctors use it to relieve pain. But the form of hypnosis practiced by these practitioners bears only a small resemblance to the nightclub hypnotist.

The American Society of Clinical Hypnosis (ASCH) is a professional organization providing training and continuing education in clinical hypnosis.

▌ What's Offered

ASCH publishes the *American Journal of Clinical Hypnosis*. Its original articles include clinical reports, case studies, abstracts, and research. The *ASCH Newsletter* brings information of upcoming events to the Society's members.

Most important to health care consumers, ASCH also provides a referral service of qualified professionals who use clinical hypnosis in their practice and will help you find one in your area.

International Medical and Dental Hypnotherapy Association
4110 Edgeland
Suite 800
Royal Oak, MI 48073
313-549-5594

▌ Background

Hypnosis is no longer the parlor trick it was once thought to be. It has many therapeutic and pain-relieving benefits just beginning to be discovered.

The International Medical and Dental Hypnotherapy Association (IMDHA) is a training and certification association of hypnotherapists. Its educational objectives are:

- ▌ To prepare the patient mentally for treatment
- ▌ To reduce panic and fear in the patient
- ▌ To teach patients self-hypnosis to control pain and to aid in healing.

▌ What's Offered

IMDHA's publication, the bimonthly ($12) *Subconsciously Speaking*, contains news of the profession and upcoming events, seminars, and workshops in the field of hypnotherapy.

The Association also maintains an international directory of hypnotherapists that is available to the general public and will help you find a professional in your area.

National Society of Hypnotherapists
2175 NW 85th
Suite 6A
Des Moines, IA 50325
515-270-2280

▌ Background

Hypnotherapy is recognized as a therapeutic modality for treating many psychological ailments, especially those involving an alteration or change in habit or behavior.

The National Society of Hypnotherapists, a professional accreditation organization of certified hypnotherapists, conducts conventions, educational seminars, and workshops in hypnotherapy.

▌ What's Offered

The Society provides training and certification in hypnotherapy. Its professional seminars and educational workshops cover such topics as:

- ▌ Hypnosis and children
- ▌ Phobias
- ▌ Addictions
- ▌ Behavioral analysis techniques
- ▌ Brain wave synchronator technology
- ▌ Whole brain study
- ▌ Forensic hypnosis.

Its quarterly publication serves as a source of continuing education in the practice of hypnotherapy.

Referrals to a professional hypnotist or hypnotherapist in your area are available.

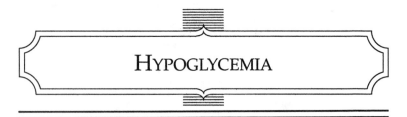

HYPOGLYCEMIA

Dr. John W. Tintera Memorial Hypoglycemia Lay Group
149 Spindle Road
Hicksville, NY 11801
516-731-3302

Contact: Elaine Arnstein

▌ Background

In spite of a diet high in sugar, many Americans suffer from chronic low blood sugar, or hypoglycemia. Almost never diagnosed as a disease, it is actually an adrenal gland metabolic dysfunction that places a strain on the entire immune system. Its symptoms are so extensive that it is often mis-diagnosed or treated as a psychosomatic, rather than a physiological, condition.

Yet, when correctly diagnosed, hypoglycemia is easily controlled and arrested, almost entirely through diet and other lifestyle changes.

The Dr. John W. Tintera Memorial Hypoglycemia Lay Group was formed to educate the general public and hypoglycemics about lifestyle changes that can prove beneficial.

▌ What's Offered

Membership ($15) includes a subscription to the Group's quarterly newsletter that includes numerous recipes and information gleaned from the scientific literature. Newsletter article topics have discussed:

▪ Mood and food

- Behavioral problems and low blood sugar
- Vitamin deficiencies
- Over-the-counter and prescription drugs
- Alcoholism—low blood sugar
- Carbohydrate values
- Stress—hypoadrenocorticism.

Hypoglycemia Association, Inc.
18008 New Hampshire Avenue
Box 165
Ashton, MD 20861
202-544-4044

▌ Background

The Hypoglycemia Association is an organization of people suffering from blood sugar problems. Concerned primarily with promoting information to both its members and the general public on managing disturbed blood sugar with dietary elimination and stress management, its focus is on self-help.

▌ What's Offered

Monthly meetings are held in the Washington, D.C. area and usually have a guest speaker who talks on a particular health matter and then takes questions from the audience.

A bimonthly newsletter is sent to members across the country and is included in the $15 yearly membership fee. Its purpose is to keep everyone concerned about blood sugar problems and informed of what's going on in the field. This one- to four-page newsletter's short, easy-to-understand articles are devoted to providing information on managing blood sugar problems. Regular features of the bulletin include letters from readers (with answers from specialists), health information from other organizations, and reviews of publications dealing with prevention as well as treatment. Some recent topics covered include:

- Adrenal glands—how they affect blood sugar
- Energy and diet
- Resources for further information on blood sugar ailments.

Reprints of all the hundreds of articles from back issues are provided in a list and are available for a nominal charge.

Academy for Guided Imagery
P.O. Box 2070
Mill Valley, CA 94942
415-389-9324
415-389-9342 (fax)

▌ Background

Guided imagery uses hypnosis and relaxation techniques to promote physical and psychological well-being through evoking the
positive self-awareness, autonomy, and personal empowerment of
patients.

Founded in 1988, the Academy for Guided Imagery (AGI) is
a training ground for professional clinicians and other health care
practioners in imagery therapies.

▌ What's Offered

AGI provides both certified training for the professional and information for the general public on imagery and imagery-related
approaches to therapy and healing. Training workshops, which
also include a great deal of information from which an interested
layperson might benefit, available on audio tapes, include:

- Pain control—imagery and biofeedback techniques
- Psychoneuroimmunology—imagery therapies
- Self-healing
- Depression
- Eating disorders
- Relaxation skills and exercises

■ Imagery techniques
■ Stress management.

Self-help books for the general public currently include:

■ *Free Yourself from Pain*
■ *Healing Yourself.*

The Academy sells a nationwide members directory, which is sure to include several practitioners using guided imagery in your area.

American Imagery Institute
P.O. Box 13453
Milwaukee, WI 53213
414-781-4045

■ Background

The use of mental imagery in healing has a place in many cultures. In the past few years modern scientific research has confirmed that emotional, psychological, and physiological changes can be effected through mental imagery.

The American Imagery Institute (AII) was formed to promote the use of imagery techniques for health care professionals. A secondary purpose is to provide a means of training to interested professionals and lay individuals to learn about the uses and benefits of guided imagery.

■ What's Offered

Through its catalogue, the Institute offers many books and audio tapes and conducts workshops on mental imagery and related

topics. Many books and workshop proceedings are for professionals in the field. But careful scrutiny will reveal enough of interest
for the individual. Some topics discussed in its publications and at
past conferences are:

- Mind–body identity
- Imagery and neural activity
- Psychosomatic illness
- Chinese medicine
- Focusing techniques
- Biofeedback and self-regulation
- Imagination and healing.

INCONTINENCE

Help for Incontinent People
P.O. Box 544
Union, SC 29397
803-579-7900
800-BLADDER (hotline)
803-579-7902 (fax)

Contact: Katherine F. Jeter, Executive Director

∎ Background

Despite the rise of incontinence, fewer than 3% of the physicians asked by their patients about this problem initiate any treatment at all, relegating their patients to "one of the inevitable problems of old age." Nothing can be further from the truth. Incontinence is neither inevitable with old age nor untreatable.

Help for Incontinent People (HIP) was founded to help the incontinent and their families to manage or satisfactorily cure incontinence.

∎ What's Offered

HIP's quarterly ($5) *HIP Report* contains numerous articles on such topics as:

- ∎ Pelvic exercises—bladder control
- ∎ Stress
- ∎ Surgery
- ∎ Embarrassment
- ∎ Products and aids

- Cure—surgery, medication
- Intestinal cystitis
- Bedwetting
- Diet and exercise—effects on incontinence.

HIP also has a number of pamphlets, audio tapes, and videos available for sale. In addition, HIP sells a resource guide of additional products and services for the incontinent and maintains a professionally staffed toll-free hotline to answer questions.

Simon Foundation
P.O. Box 815
Wilmette, IL 60091
800-23SIMON
708-864-9758 (fax)

Contact: Cheryle B. Gartley

▌ Background

Many health problems are never discussed and remain in the closet because of fear or embarrassment. One such problem is incontinence: loss of bladder control. It's a serious problem to more than 12 million Americans.

The Simon Foundation endeavors to help the incontinent and their families to manage or satisfactorily cure this problem.

▌ What's Offered

A $15 membership will get you the Foundation's four-page quarterly, *The Informer*. Each issue is devoted to a single topic. Regular features include readers' letters and product reviews. Some recent topics on incontinence have included:

- Age and incontinence
- Products
- Enlarged prostate in older men
- Intermittent catheterization
- Operations and stress in females
- Talking to your doctor
- Urinary tract infections.

A book on managing the problem and an extensive video program produced by the University of Manchester's (England) Department of Geriatric Medicine are available.

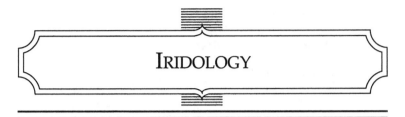

IRIDOLOGY

National Iridology Research Association
P.O. Box 33637
Seattle, WA 98133
206-363-5980

Contact: William Caradonna

▌ Background

The eyes are the windows of the soul. But are they also windows to disease diagnosis? Iridology says yes.

Iridology is the practice of diagnosing the ills of the body through the study of the iris of the eye. More specifically, the patterns of the eye's blood vessels, eye color and eye hue are said to serve as indicators of the specific diseases and ailments of the body.

The National Iridology Research Association serves as the accrediting and educational agency for iridologists and as an educational forum to educate the general public and other health care professionals.

▌ What's Offered

Iridology isn't much practiced or widely accepted as valid in the United States although it is practiced in many European countries.

For $35 you will get a year's membership in the Association and a subscription to their quarterly journal, *Iridology Review*. Past issues of the magazine have discussed such topics as:

- ▌ News affecting the profession

- Herbs and nutrition to supplement iridology
- Iridology and homeopathy
- Applied kinesiology testing
- Digestion and iridology
- Diagnostic techniques.

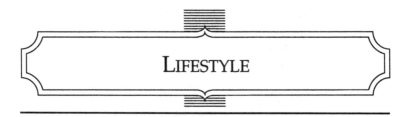

LIFESTYLE

American Journal of Health Promotion
1812 South Rochester Road
Suite 200
Birmingham, MI 48307
313-650-9600
313-650-9602 (fax)

▌ Background

Forty-eight percent of all deaths in the United States are the result of poor lifestyle habits. Is this a new finding? Hardly. It was reported by the Centers for Disease Control over a decade ago. Only recently has the death rate begun to drop and has "wellness" become a watchword for the fashionable.

The peer-reviewed *American Journal of Health Promotion* is a bimonthly ($49.50) devoted to promoting positive lifestyle changes. The publisher defines this journal by defining health promotion as "the science and art of helping people change their lifestyle to move toward a state of optimal health."

▌ What's Offered

The Journal's approximately 100 pages of technical information is divided into 23 areas of editorial interest, and then grouped into five further sections: intervention, strategy, application, research, and information exchange. Monthly features include data case studies, literature and product reviews, abstracts, and database critiques. Recently published article topics are:

▪ Ethnicity and lifestyle health risk

■ Adult fitness program components
■ Spiritual health promotion
■ Worksite health programs
■ Employee stress.

Conferences for professionals are sponsored on a regular basis where papers on clinical practices and health promotion are presented.

Balance
Balance Publications
359 Walden Green
Branford, CT 06405
203-481-3661

■ Background

Balance, published bimonthly ($18), calls itself "the magazine for wholistic lifestyles."

■ What's Offered

This 48-page magazine features short, pithy articles written by well-known experts and journalists on health, self-esteem, human potential, and physical fitness. Recent articles have covered such topics as:

■ Yoga and negativity
■ Channeling
■ Organic and biodynamic gardening
■ Fitness.

EastWest
East West Partners
17 Station Street
Box 1200
Brookline, MA 02147
617-232-1000

▌ Background

EastWest: The Journal of Natural Health & Living is a slick, full-color, 100-page plus monthly ($24) magazine providing information and promoting and encouraging alternative lifestyles and ways of thinking.

▌ What's Offered

EastWest is devoted to giving practical advice on alternative medicine, lifestyle changes, whole foods and cooking, women's health, and diet and nutrition. The articles are written by experts in the field, on a variety of topics, and almost always include information on where to get further information: books, organizations, and experts. Recent article topics have included:

- Surviving with AIDS
- Organic agriculture
- Back massage—pain relief and muscle relaxation
- Medical freedom of choice
- Headache relief—herbal products and nontoxic therapies
- Alternative M.D.'s—guidelines for choosing one
- Radon—testing for it
- Osteopathy—what it is and how to find an osteopath
- Medical and health software review.

A large variety of books on alternative health—treatment, prevention, diet, and cooking, as well as books on practical ecology and animal rights are sold through a yearly catalogue.

Lifestyle Medicine Institute
11538 Anderson Street
P.O. Box 474
Loma Linda, CA 92354
714-796-7676

▌ Background

If proof were needed that lifestyle can do more for health than anything medicine can do, look at the successes of the Ornish programs and the Pritikin Centers for people who have had atherosclerosis. Radical changes in diet, exercise, and stress reduction have not only controlled heart disease but have reversed its damage.

The Lifestyle Medicine Institute (LMI), founded by Dr. Hans Diehl, former head of Research and Health Education at the Pritikin Longevity Center, focuses entirely on health and disease prevention through personal self-help.

▌ What's Offered

The LMI offers a 16-page, bimonthly ($12) newsletter, *Lifeline Health Letter*. The articles are short and to the point and offer practical tips for health through personal change. Recent article topics have been:

- Heart disease—prevention from childhood
- Hypoxic diseases
- Meat consumption—personal and environmental health
- Weight loss—meal planning
- Colon cancer—high-fat diet risk
- Breast cancer—low-fat diet prevention
- Fast food—fat percentage analysis.

In addition to the newsletter, the Institute offers several books, audio tapes, and videos prepared by its staff. All follow much of the Pritikin philosophy of a low-fat, vegetarian diet and exercise.

National Wellness Institute, Inc.
University of Wisconsin
South Hall
1319 Fremont Street
Stevens Point, WI 54481
715-346-2172

▮ Background

Organizations both large and small are feeling the financial pinch of increasing costs associated with medical benefits for their employees. Many have decided that prevention will not only benefit their profit margins but also make for a healthier and more productive work force.

The stated mission of the National Wellness Institute (NWI) Inc. is:

- To assist organizations in their wellness programs
- To provide and develop such programs
- To be a resource center for wellness information
- To conduct research itself and disseminate the research results of others.

▮ What's Offered

With an eye more toward organizations than individuals, the NWI currently offers training to professionals and a variety of products: audio tapes, videos, computer health assessment, and evaluation software; consulting services to other organizations with wellness programs, and their quarterly, *Wellness Management*.

The NWI also promotes and holds several major conferences on wellness programs.

New York Open Center, Inc.
83 Spring Street
New York, NY 10012
212-219-2527

▌ Background

The New York Open Center, Inc. is much like the Omega Institute discussed below. But instead of a health retreat, this organization is more of an open university or adult education center.

▌ What's Offered

Unfortunately, all courses are held in New York. Some are all-day workshops; others are single evening classes. Many ongoing classes have up to six sessions. Peruse the Center's catalogue listing of alternative health courses and workshops and you will be sure to find something that interests you:

- Nontoxic homes
- Meditation techniques
- Building and restoring self-esteem
- Feldenkrais method
- Self-reflexology
- Seasonal health
- Shiatsu treatments
- Alexander technique.

Omega Institute for Holistic Studies
Lake Drive
Rural Delivery 2
Box 377
Rhinebeck, NY 12572
914-338-6030
914-338-0474 (fax)

■ Background

Strictly speaking, The Omega Institute is not an alernative health care resource, yet it belongs in this book of alternative health care resources.

Omega is a health retreat cum-New age weekend workshop and learning center. And, because many of the workshops, seminars, and courses will provide short, informative introductions to alternative healing modalities and psychological systems for sociopersonal problems, I have included it.

■ What's Offered

If you write, telephone, or fax, a near-100-page color catalogue will be in your mailbox within a few days. In it you will find dozens and dozens of summer programs (and winter weekends) on every conceivable psychological and psychophysical approach to well-being imaginable.

Health seminars run the gamut from body-centered approaches to cross-cultural healing, to sports and fitness. Examples include:

■ Hellerwork
■ Feldenkrais method
■ Myotherapy
■ Qi gong
■ Traditional Chinese medicine.

Psychological courses run the range from personal growth to addiction to intuitive development. Some topics included are:

- High-performance learning
- Compulsive eating
- Focusing
- Self-esteem.

Total Health
6001 Topanga Canyon Boulevard
Suite 300
Woodland Hills, CA 91367
818-887-6484

▌Background

Many magazines are available on health and a natural lifestyle. Most are similar to each other. The stories tend to be on similar topics. The recipes and seasonal topics have a familiar look to them. This is not a criticism; reading several articles or books on a topic will always aid understanding.

Total Health joins this group. It focuses on holistic health, nutrients, recipes for a healthier life, environmental concerns, and spiritual connectedness.

▌What's Offered

Total Health, a 62-page, full-color, bimonthly ($12), contains regular columns on skin care, exercising, travel, herbalism, body–mind connection, and book, audio tape, and video reviews. Many articles are written by recognized health authorities. Most are physicians or other health care professionals. The articles are all literate and

free from jargon and stress the practical rather than the theoretical.
Sample topics from several recent issues include:

▪ Nutrition—digestion
▪ Gum disease—natural prevention
▪ Exercising—bad knees
▪ Recipes—vegetarian barbecue
▪ Enzymes—free radical and antigen protection
▪ Garlic—anti-infection capabilities.

Further Resources
see also all resources under PREVENTION
Bestways
Cardiac Alert
Institute for the Study of Human Knowledge
Macrobiotics Today
Natural Health
Natural Lifestyle and Your Health
Natural Living Newsletter
Solstice
Spectrum
Today's Living

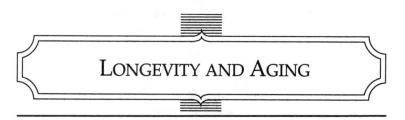

LONGEVITY AND AGING

Alliance for Aging Research
2021 K Street, NW
Suite 305
Washington, DC 20006
202-293-2856

▌ Background

The Alliance for Aging Research provides information on aging to the general public and seeks to increase the priority of age-related research on health.

▌ What's Offered

Conferences on aging and their audio tape transcripts are available, along with the quarterly *Alliance Reports*, all sold to raise money for research. The newsletter contains articles on current legislature, women's health, diseases of the elderly, and scientific findings of new research. Information in the newsletter and that presented at conferences stresses independent living and self-help with an emphasis on the practical.

American Aging Association
University of Nebraska Medical Center
600 South 42nd Street
Omaha, NE 68198-4635
402-559-4416

Attn.: Dr. Denham Harman

▌ Background

By the time you finish reading this you will be about a minute older. Aging itself—the significant decrease in functionality—is more important in life extension than almost anything else.

For example, if all cancers were miraculously cured, the average lifespan would be extended less than 23 months. If cardiovascular diseases were suddenly wiped out, the average lifespan would be increased by about seven years. But if we could slow down the aging process, you and I might live another 20 to 40 years.

The American Aging Association is dedicated to supporting biomedical research in human longevity, specifically:

- ▌ To determine why we age
- ▌ To find practical ways to slow down the aging process
- ▌ To educate the public and keep health care professionals informed about biomedical aging research.

▌ What's Offered

A $25 membership supports research and gives you a subscription to *Age News*, AAAs four-page quarterly newsletter. In each issue you will find current research findings in age-related biomedical research, such as:

- ▌ Potassium and aging humans
- ▌ Physical fitness and mortality
- ▌ Menopause risk factors for coronary heart disease.

American Federation for Aging Research, Inc.
725 Park Avenue
New York, NY 10021
212-570-2090
212-570-2496 (fax)

Contact: Harold Epstein, Executive Vice President

▌ Background

Each of us is growing older. Many of us are living longer. In fact, the fastest growing age group is that of 85 and older.

The American Federation for Aging Research (AFAR), Inc. promotes support and provides the research funds for biomedical research on aging.

▌ What's Offered

A contribution to support their research will get you a subscription to their quarterly six-page newsletter, the *AFAR Newsletter*. In it you'll find news of current grants made to researchers and the results of research and clinical studies done by past recipients.

American Longevity Association
1000 West Carson Street
Box 22
Torrance, CA 90509
213-544-7057

Contact: Dr. Robert J. Morin

▌ Background

The American Longevity Association, whose scientific and advisory boards consist of six Nobel laureates, is devoted to presenting

practical information to the layperson who wants to extend his or
her life.

▌ What's Offered

Although the Association no longer publishes its newsletter, *Longevity Letter* on a regular basis, a large number of recent back issues
are available. Considering the preeminence of its boards, they may
be worthwhile investigating. Each 12-page issue consists of a comprehensive summary of the latest research presented in a practical,
ready-to-use manner. Also included is a comprehensive reference
list that you can use for follow-up research. Topics presented have
included:

- ▌ Food restriction—lifespan extension
- ▌ Vitamin C—age-related illnesses
- ▌ Ginseng—effect on aging immune system
- ▌ Alcohol and brain damage
- ▌ Relaxation—blood pressure
- ▌ Cooking and mutagens

Durk Pearson & Sandy Shaw's *Life Extension Newsletter*
P.O. Box 92996
Los Angeles, CA 90009

▌ Background

Although we will all die someday, we all want to live as long as
we can provided that life is vital. That is the subject of the booming
life extension business.

Durk Pearson and Sandy Shaw, the authors of *Life Extension*,
may be able to take much of the credit for that bonanza. Their
monthly ($34.95) newsletter carries on their high-tech approach to
health and longevity.

▌ What's Offered

Pearson and Shaw's approach is not that of nature, holism, and unconventional therapies. Instead, they focus on the leading edge of what's new in current scientific research on aging and life extension. They believe that nutrients and pharmaceuticals can extend your life without the need for the restrictions imposed by vegetarianism and most other alternative health researchers.

Their monthly newsletter regularly covers the following topics:

- ▌ Immune system improvement
- ▌ Losing body fat
- ▌ Free-radical antioxidants
- ▌ Health book reviews
- ▌ FDA policies
- ▌ Reviews of scientific research studies
- ▌ Answers to readers' questions.

Forefront—Health Investigations
MegaHealth Society
P.O. Box 60637
Palo Alto, CA 94306
408-733-2010

Contact: Steven William Fowkes, Editor

▌ Background

The MegaHealth Society publishes *Forefront—Health Investigations* ($18) six times a year, along with a number of books on special topics of importance in longevity and health. The uniqueness of this newsletter is due to its concentrating on antiaging information, metabolic balancing through pH, and BHT information and viral diseases.

▌ What's Offered

Life extension, combined with biological technology, is the thrust of this newsletter. All articles on longevity are literate and very detailed without being complicated, contain much background technical information, are practical (formulations and amounts) in their application, and include extensive references. Recent issues have included articles on:

- Candida albicans—possible treatments
- Activated charcoal as an internal body detoxifier—how much and how often
- AIDS—new research and treatment possibilities
- Measuring your biological age—self-testing
- Brain melatonin—understanding the brain's cycles
- Selenium deficiency—what harm it can do
- Hypericin—St. John's Wort derivative and antiviral activity in AIDS
- Allergies and hyperactivity—food and nutrients
- Understanding the immune system.

Several books, the complete set of back issues of the journal, and reports on a variety of subjects are also sold, including:

- Life extension—nutrients to live longer
- Herpes—BHT as a treatment
- Infant mortality
- Metabolic balancing—acid/alkaline foods.

Life Extension Foundation
2490 Griffin Road
Fort Lauderdale, FL 33312
800-841-5433

█ Background

How much longer could you live if you did not fall prey to the most common degenerative and chronic diseases? While scientists still differ as to the precise age, most agree that human beings would live at least 120 years.

The Life Extension Foundation believes that aging itself makes us more susceptible to the common diseases that kill the majority of us. But most importantly, it believes that there is, and funds research for, a "cure" for or at least a way of controlling aging.

█ What's Offered

Membership in the Foundation entitles you to two monthly newsletters, *Life Extension Report* and *Life Extension Update*. Both discuss in short articles of a few paragraphs to two pages the latest research on the benefits of nutrients on life extension and disease prevention and efforts to prevent aging and to rejuvenate the aged. Recent topics discussed are:

- █ Mineral supplementation recommendations—magnesium, potassium, calcium
- █ Cataracts—antioxidant protection
- █ Chromium picolinate—lean body mass
- █ Carotenoids
- █ Gingivitis
- █ Weight-loss therapies.

All the nutrients discussed in the newsletters, as well as many others, are available at discount prices to Foundation members from its catalogue. Several books and audio tapes on life extension and products for longevity are also available.

Additional benefits include a pharmaceutical hotline, information on obtaining pharamaceuticals that are not yet approved from foreign countries, and a nationwide list of physicians who are knowledgeable about life extension and clinics providing unapproved therapies for cancer, AIDS, Alzheimer's, and other disorders.

Longevity
Longevity International, Ltd.
1965 Broadway
New York, NY 10023-5965
212-496-6100

▌Background

Longevity seems more and more to be the latest craze among craze-hungry Americans. Televison, radio, news articles, and human-interest stories revolve around the long life rather than the good life.

Now, along comes a magazine, *Longevity*, devoted exclusively to the long, and very good, life.

▌What's Offered

This 100-page, monthly ($17.97), four-color magazine is put out by the publishers of *Penthouse* so be forewarned: Sleek, beautiful, bare bodies seem to be a main ingredient of the long life as prescribed by its editors.

Nonetheless, the articles and stories are thoroughly researched, well-documented, and run from the theoretical to the very practical. There are also regular features on health news, natural herbal cures for common complaints, health and prevention advice, antiaging news, and the usual bill of fare. However, this is not an exclusively alternative health care or prevention magazine; enough solid information is included in every issue to be included here. Recent topics covered have been:

- Rating fat-free ice creams
- Immunity cocktails—immune-stimulating drugs and cancer remission
- Self-acupressure—how to do it, where to do it, what to do it for
- Privately funded life extension research
- Mind-stimulating-cum-relating machines—electronic workouts for the brain
- Cosmetic surgery—dangers and warnings
- Harassing alternative physicians
- Antioxidants—recipes for summer desserts
- Breast implants—risks, dangers.

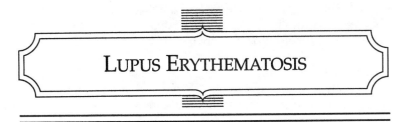

Lupus Erythematosis

Lupus Foundation of America, Inc.
1717 Massachusetts Avenue, NW
Suite 203
Washington, DC 20036
202-328-4550

Contact: Virginia T. Ladd, R.T.

▌ Background

Lupus erythematosis is a chronic inflammatory disease of the connective tissues striking a person's immune system. More than half a million men, women, and children suffer from lupus, with 50,000 more affected every year. Although there is no cure for lupus at present, several treatments are available for its control.

The Lupus Foundation of America (LFA), Inc. is devoted to making the public aware of lupus, and provides support for lupus sufferers and their families through its 100-plus local chapters.

▌ What's Offered

While some information and a list of local chapters is available from the LFA—including a short list of books and monographs you can purchase—it is your local chapter that will prove most helpful.

Within a week of writing or telephoning LFA, your own state's Lupus Foundation will send you an information packet. It contains details about lupus, relates how lifestyle, diet, and medication can control it, tell you of local meetings in your immediate neighborhood, and includes a sample copy of the local newsletter.

A $10 membership fee makes you a member of your state chapter and one of its local support groups. It and its local affiliates serve as support groups, and their newsletters normally convey information about upcoming activities, news of members, and articles on self-help and care.

Many state-level groups sell books, audio tapes, and videos on lupus. Recent articles from several state organization newsletters include:

- Women and osteoporosis
- Headaches and lupus
- Effect of ultraviolet light
- Effect of drugs and summer sun
- Dietary guidelines for lupus sufferers
- Dry-eye syndrome treatment and its prevention.

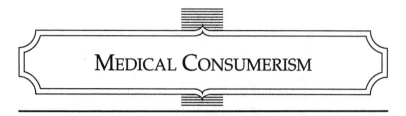

MEDICAL CONSUMERISM

Center for Medical Consumers
237 Thompson Street
New York, NY 10012
212-674-7105

▌ Background

Is there a time of day that a health cum-medical show isn't on cable television? Are we getting too much health information, or just noise masquerading as knowledge?

The Center for Medical Consumers (CMC) thinks that whatever information about health is getting through speaks with a single voice: that of organized medicine. Conversely, the CMC believes that:

- Understanding your illness and its causes will help you better choose a treatment and contribute to your healing
- You have a legal right to all information about your medical history.

▌ What's Offered

HealthFacts, the Center's monthly ($18) newsletter, is charged with the task of helping you determine the need, risks, and effectiveness of many common medical procedures and showing you all treatment options, including nonmedical ones, for illnesses. Each issue discusses one topic in depth, presenting resources for follow-up. Past issues have covered both common, degenerative, and chronic conditions such as:

- Anxiety disorders

- Light in healing
- Over-the-counter cold remedies
- Mammography screening for women in their 40s
- Diagnostic test guidelines
- Quick cholesterol testing
- Treating pain
- Medical and dental X-rays.

The Center's extensive library of more than 1500 books and journals is available for reference. A substantial amount of alternative approaches to health and disease is on file in that library.

Doctor's People Newsletter
1578 Sherman Avenue
Suite 318
Evanston, IL 60201

Background

Many critics of conventional medicine are themselves physicians. Dr. Robert S. Mendelsohn was such a critic.

As part of the effort to educate consumers about his concerns he published a monthly newsletter, *The People's Doctor*. After his recent untimely death, it is being continued as the *Doctor's People Newsletter*.

What's Offered

A $24 subscription to this eight-page, monthly newsletter, written by doctors who are on its advisory board, will allow you to keep up with a variety of maverick opinions on many health topics you may never even have heard of. Topics have included:

- Mandatory measles immunization—safety and efficacy
- AIDS and the smallpox vaccine

- Down's syndrome and Feldene
- Kidney and liver diseases—silver nitrate cholesterol medicine
- Arthritis drugs—oraflex et al.
- Blood transfusions
- Hypoglycemia and ulcerative colitis
- Steroid drugs.

People's Medical Society
462 Walnut Street
Allentown, PA 18102
215-770-1670

Background

Alternative health care not only means nonconventional therapies and prevention, it also means alternative ways of informing yourself about orthodox medical treatment and of looking at any therapy or medical advice offered to you by a health care practitioner.

The 80,000 member People's Medical Society (PMS) seeks to get health and medical information into the hands of consumers and to make America's medical establishment more responsive to its customers' needs.

What's Offered

Joining the PMS ($15) will entitle you to receive its monthly newsletter. In it you will find short, lively, easy-to-understand articles on choosing a doctor or specialist, case histories of people who have successfully fought for their medical rights, exposés of unethical and incompetent practitioners, and how to avoid unnecessary treatment.

There are also countless health bulletins, medical information packets, books, special publications, bibliographies, and illness updates available at discount prices.

Public Voice
1001 Connecticut Avenue, NW
Suite 522
Washington, DC 20036
202-659-5930

▌ Background

We are all dependent upon others for the quality and safety of our food. Almost none of us grows all our own food or picks it from a tree or roots it out of the ground from soil that is entirely free of pesticides and herbicides. Few of us even buy our food directly from the farmer. In fact, whether we live in the city, suburbs, or even on a farm, nearly all of us get our food from the supermarket.

Whether we like this or not, this makes food as much a part of government as defense. Public Voice acts as a consumer advocate in the areas of food, health, and nutrition.

▌ What's Offered

Public Voice, aside from holding food policy conferences and workshops, publishes many reports and books on:

- Agricultural policy—pesticides, subsidies, dairy prices
- Fish and seafood—inspection, shellfish contamination, health risks
- Food and nutrition—biotechnology, dietary fat reduction, empty calories, food hazards
- Rural poverty—infant health, migrant workers
- School lunch—reducing fat
- Women's health issues—contraception.

Second Opinion
P.O. Box 84908
Phoenix, AZ 85071-9967
800-528-0559

Background

Iatrogenesis: You probably have never heard of this killer of millions. Yet each year it injures and kills thousands of people. What is it? Iatrogenesis is injury or death due to physicians—their procedures, treatments, surgical proceedings, and drugs. It's not that a doctor means to do harm, but it happens every day.

To diminish your chances of becoming a victim of iatrogenesis you need information, information from a different perspective: another opinion of what to do and perhaps more important of what not to do. That's the purpose of *Second Opinion*.

What's Offered

This monthly newsletter offers information on useless medical treatments, including many widely practiced surgical techniques, tests, and prescription drugs. More importantly, it presents information on many safe treatments that have been proven to heal. Topics that have been covered in several past issues include:

- Vaccines—problems of contamination
- Fluoridation—links to illnesses
- Dentistry—mercury fillings
- Medical tests—doctors and the labs they own
- Aspirin—dangers
- Alzheimer's—the risks
- High blood pressure—inexpensive cure
- Questioning your doctor—what he or she doesn't want you to ask.

Further Resources
National Health Federation

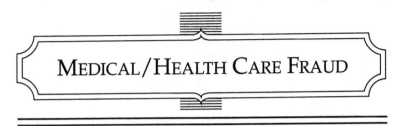

MEDICAL/HEALTH CARE FRAUD

Health Letter
Public Citizen Health Research Group
2000 P Street, NW
Washington, DC 20036
202-872-0320

Contact: Dr. Sidney M. Wolfe, Editor

▌ Background

A monthly newsletter ($14.95), *Health Letter* informs its readers of
medical news that affects the treatment they receive from physicians. Part of a Ralph Nader consumer advocacy group, the staff
of the Public Citizen Health Research Group often files Freedom of
Information Act law suits to get the medical and hospital data they
report.

▌ What's Offered

The newsletter does not cover topics relating to what you should
do to promote your own health. Instead, in an entirely confronta-
tional manner, it is devoted to reporting news of the medical
establishment, news that the medical establishment often does not
want reported. Recent topics covered include:

▪ Physicians whose practices have been barred or who have
   financial ties to products they prescribe
▪ Questionable and dangerous medical devices not yet banned
   by the FDA

- Best and worst hospitals for treatment based on the hospitals' own mortality rates
- The dangers of both over-the-counter and prescription drugs
- Findings of costly surgical practices and therapies that are unnecessary or dangerous
- Abuse and overprescribing of anitbiotics for bacterial infections.

Further Resources
Doctor's People Newsletter

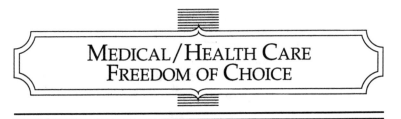

MEDICAL/HEALTH CARE FREEDOM OF CHOICE

Association of Concerned Citizens for Preventive Medicine
415-B McArthur Avenue
Ottawa
Ontario, Canada K1K 1G5
613-749-1002

▍ Background

Medical freedom of choice is as much a problem to our neighbor to the north, Canada, as it is to us in the United States. The availability of alternative therapies and the right to refuse certain types of treatment are at risk in Canada.

The Association of Concerned Citizens for Preventive Medicine (ACCPM) focuses on disseminating information on preventive medicine and the encouragement of research into therapies and lifestyle changes that are more preventive than curative.

▍ What's Offered

A $25 contribution will entitle you to receive a year's subscription to ACCPM's 12-page, bimonthly newsletter. Most topics are related to Canadian medicine but much is directly applicable in America. Topics discussed in the last few issues are:

- ▍ Food irradiation
- ▍ Chelation therapy
- ▍ AIDS
- ▍ Chiropractry
- ▍ Traditional Chinese medicine and acupuncture

∎ Vaccination and immunization.

Many short features will give you information about Canadian organizations devoted to preventive health care and nutrition and the health risks with standard medical practices.

Choice
Committee for Freedom of Choice in Medicine, Inc.
1180 Walnut Avenue
Chula Vista, CA 92011
619-429-8200

∎ Background

It is clear that although America may be the freest country in the world, that freedom does not extend to health care.

Choice, a 40-page, quarterly published by the lobbying group Committee for Freedom of Choice in Medicine, Inc., is also associated with American Biologics, an alternative health care clinic using a variety of metabolic therapies to treat degenerative and chronic diseases.

∎ What's Offered

The articles are written by professionals associated with the clinic and present news of alternative therapies. Many of the topics discuss the specific therapies of American Biologics and are presented in a scholarly manner with references for follow-up study. Some topics from recent issues include:

∎ Diet immunity connection
∎ Dioxychlor—live cell therapy
∎ Anticholesterol—science or scam?
∎ Homeopathy—AIDS, cancer

■ AIDS—iatrogenic connection.

Additionally, many articles discuss the erosion of medical freedom of choice and the abuses of the orthodox medical establishment.

Citizens for Alternative Health Care
15611 Bel-Red Road
Building A
Bellevue, WA 98008
206-869-7767

▌ Background

In 1989, a study showed that every year more than 73,000 elderly died and 1.9 million Americans were hospitalized from taking too much or the wrong drug prescribed by their physicians. The U.S. Congress's Office of Technology Assessment said in September 1978, that only between 10% and 20% of all medical procedures were shown to be effective by a controlled study and trial. The *Wall Street Journal* reported in June 1989 that repeated public opinion polls always show more and more Americans "unhappy with the nation's health care system."

The all-too-familiar, not-too-surprising prescription from government is more of the same: Throw more of the taxpayer's dollars at it. Those dollars, though, will only go for more of the same—more pharmaceuticals, more surgical procedures. Nothing will be spent on prevention; nothing on alternative therapies.

The stated purpose of the Citizens for Alternative Health Care (CAHC) is to make sure that there are no legal barriers preventing physicians and patients from choosing their own therapies. In the case of CAHC, those therapies are natural and non-invasive.

▌ What's Offered

CAHC pursues the legislative and legal route to preserve medical freedom of choice. Personal lobbying, telephone and letter campaigns, and testimony before legislative bodies are the routes they use.

A four-page, monthly newsletter discusses promising alternative therapies.

Coalition for Alternatives in Nutrition and Healthcare, Inc.
P.O. Box B-12
Richlandtown, PA 18955
215-346-8461

▌ Background

It's an old saw that you lose something when someone takes it away from you a little bit at a time. Little by little what you once had is taken away from you until it's all gone. So it is with anything you fear to lose, but fail to safeguard. So it is with freedom of choice in health care.

The Coalition for Alternatives in Nutrition and Healthcare (CANAH), Inc., supports the adoption of a health care rights amendment and provides a series of brochures and pamphlets promoting this viewpoint and showing the efficacy of alternative health care.

▌ What's Offered

A slew of free brochures on the proposed amendment are yours for writing to CANAH. An additional set of health-related pamphlets and books are sold to support their work. These include information on:

∎ Evaluation of the American Medical Association as a doctor's trade union
∎ Double-blind study evaluation
∎ Food irradiation fact sheets
∎ Antilicensing documentation packets
∎ Vitamin mineral reprints
∎ Formaldehyde dangers
∎ Immunization hazards
∎ Benefits of nutrition research.

Foundation for the Advancement of Innovative Medicine
P.O. Box 338
Kinderhook, NY 12106
800-462-3246

∎ Background

Do you believe in medical freedom of choice? Do you want to have the right to choose an unconventional, alternative therapy for an illness? Would you like your medical insurance to cover preventive therapies and treatments that have shown promise but do not include drugs or surgery?

If you answered yes to any of those questions and believe them important, the Foundation for the Advancement of Innovative Medicine (FAIM) may be worth your while. Its purpose is to protect your right to choose a treatment or therapy that is outside of conventional medicine, but has been shown to have clinical benefits. In other words, to assure your medical freedom of choice.

∎ What's Offered

The $25 membership will entitle you to a subscription to *Innovation*, FAIMs quarterly journal. It serves as a forum where professional health care practitioners and interested individuals can exchange ideas and views on assuring both freedom of choice and guaranteeing medical insurance reimbursement for alternative and complementary treatments. Articles on alternative health care systems are also a regular feature.

Yearly symposia featuring leading alternative health care practitioners are sponsered through FAIM's auspices.

A membership roster is available that includes many leading health care practitioners using alternative therapies, and issues of *Innovation* often contain a list of professionals (many of whom include the use of alternative therapies) in private practice.

Independent Citizens Research Foundation for the Study of Degenerative Diseases, Inc.

P.O. Box 97
Ardsley, NY 10502
914-478-1862

Contact: Dorothea P. Seeber

▌ Background

It's a tired, old adage that the industrial era is dead and we live in the information age. But in spite of the information overload that bombards us daily, many people feel that it is altogether too one-sided. That, of course, depends on which side your beliefs are buttered on.

The stated purpose of the Independent Citizens Research Foundation (ICRF) for the Study of Degenerative Diseases, Inc. is to provide information on a variety of health-related subjects that aren't being offered elsewhere.

▌ What's Offered

You cannot join the ICRF. There is no membership in the ICRF. Its policies are that doctors have the right to choose what they consider the best therapy for their patients, that medical researchers have the right to pursue what they feel is the best treatment without harassment, and that patients have a right to request their therapy of choice.

The Foundation publishes a wide variety of medical and environmental health information in newsletters and bulletins for which they would appreciate a contribution from the recipients. The material is well-documented and scholarly without being technical, and thoroughly supports a particular viewpoint. Recent topics include:

- Nuclear safety
- Food irradiation
- Immune system and wellness
- Stressful lifestyles and heart disease
- Faith and therapy.

ICRF also publishes and makes available an extensive series of reprints of the writings and broadcasts of Carlton Fredericks.

National Health Federation
P.O. Box 688
212 Foothill Boulevard
Monrovia, CA 91017-9970
818-357-2181
818-359-8334

∎ Background

Every liberty, every freedom, every right is always in danger, even in America.

At the country's founding, Dr. Benjamin Rush, a signer of the Declaration of Independence, warned the Sons of Liberty: "Unless we put medical freedom into the Constitution, the time will come when medicine will organize itself into an undercover dictatorship. . . . To restrict the art of healing to one class of men and deny equal privileges to others will constitute the Bastille of medical science."

The National Health Federation (NHF) is a grass-roots, nonprofit, health-rights organization devoted to "the civil liberty of freedom of choice in matters of personal health."

∎ What's Offered

A $36 membership fee entitles you to *Health Freedom News* that serves as the organization's public voice.

A variety of books on disease prevention, nutrition, diet, and alternative treatments for diseases are offered for sale, and several conventions and seminars on a variety of alternative health-related topics are held every year.

Patient Rights Legal Action Fund

202 West 78th Street
Suite 3E
New York, NY 10024
212-580-8983
212-580-9570

Contact: Avis Long, Coordinator

Background

It is believed by many that the U.S. Food and Drug Administration
(FDA) protects the public from medical fraud and quackery, ap-
proves and monitors pharmaceuticals, and makes sure that no
company or professional practitioner makes a medical claim for a
product or therapy that cannot be substantiated.

Others, including the Patient Rights Legal Action Fund
(PRLAF), dispute this, believing that the FDA's policies and practices
serve merely to harass new and innovative treatments, and prevent
patients from choosing therapies that they have decided are best.

What's Offered

The PRLAF acts as a clearinghouse in this dispute on the side of
freedom of choice, specifically in the case of cancer patients being
forced to take the FDA to court to get the treatments they want.

To support their work, the PRLAF sells a booklet and video
on cancer treatments and political policy.

Further Resources
American Nutritionists' Association
Coalition for Alternatives in Nutrition and Healthcare, Inc.
Consumers Advocating the Legalization of Midwifery
Council for Responsible Nutrition
Foundation for Innovation in Medicine
Friends of Homebirth
Patient Advocates for Advanced Cancer Treatments, Inc.
People Against Cancer

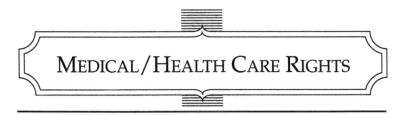

MEDICAL/HEALTH CARE RIGHTS

Committee for Truth In Psychiatry
P.O. Box 76925
Washington, DC 20013
703-979-5398

Contact: Marilyn Rice

▌ Background

An altogether too-common treatment for several psychological ailments is electric shock treatment, or Electro-Convulsive Therapy (ECT). Consisting of a series of electric shocks through the skull, it often causes epilepticlike seizures. Brain damage, severe brain trauma, and permanent memory loss is often reported even though the patient feels relaxed, calm, and comfortable for a few days to a couple of months after the treatment.

The Committee for Truth In Psychiatry (CTIP) is a grass-roots organization of former ECT patients who believe that the adverse effects and damaging results of this treatment are never told to patients and their families.

▌ What's Offered

CTIP wishes to remedy this medical situation through the use of informed consent. Informed consent means telling the prospective patient what ECT is, how it can help, and what it can do in the way of adverse side effects.

If you know of anyone contemplating ECT for themselves or a family member, contacting the CTIP may help that person make an informed choice as to whether or not to accept this form of therapy.

National Alliance For the Mentally Ill
2101 Wilson Boulevard
Suite 302
Arlington, VA 22201
703-524-7600
703-524-9094 (fax)

Contact: Laurie M. Flynn, Executive Director

▌ Background

The National Alliance For the Mentally Ill (NAMI) is a nationwide, grass-roots, self-help, support, and advocacy organization comprised of the families and friends of the mentally ill, whether psychologically or biologically based.

NAMI's primary concerns are:

- Patient and family support
- Patient advocacy
- Public education
- Research in the area of mental illness.

▌ What's Offered

Besides publishing a variety of pamphlets on many emotional ailments, each with a clear explanation of the problem, its symptoms, current treatments, and a reading list, the Alliance maintains a network of local chapters and advocacy councils. Pamphlet topics include:

- Depression and manic depression
- Schizophrenia
- Depression
- Tardive dyskinesia
- Insurance for treatment
- Panic disorder.

For $25 you will get memberships in the national group and any local one in your area that is a part of their network and a subscription to all five newsletters published by NAMI: *NAMI Advocate, The Alliance, Curriculum and Training, Forensic Monitor,* and *Sibling (and Adult Children) Bond.*

State and local groups offer family support, news of treatments, and referrals to both alternative and orthodox practitioners who have benefited their members.

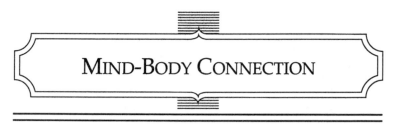

MIND-BODY CONNECTION

American Association for Therapeutic Humor
1163 Shermer Road
Northbrook, IL 60062-4538
708-291-0211

Contact: Sue Wells, Executive Director

▌ Background

It's impossible not to feel good when you're laughing. Humor, laughter, and lightheartedness all improve well-being.

The American Association for Therapeutic Humor (AATH) is devoted to making health professionals and laypersons aware of the benefits of humor as therapy. As an example, clinical studies show the many benefits of humor to include:

- Stress reduction
- Easing communication of feelings
- Improvement in circulation and digestion
- Respiratory and muscular system work-out
- Blood pressure reduction.

▌ What's Offered

A $35 membership entitles you to a subscription to AATHs six-page, bimonthly newsletter, *Laugh It Up* and a bibliography of humor in one of several areas. Recent articles in *Laugh It Up* have been on:

- Health care and humor

- Humor and personal crisis
- Jewish humor
- Humor in tough times
- Laughter and disabilities.

Each issue includes news of the Association and upcoming events.

Archaeus Project
2402 University Avenue
St. Paul, MN 55114
612-781-5012
612-641-0153 (fax)

Contact: Dennis Stillings, Project Director

Background

The Archaeus Project believes that the mind and emotions play not only a part in physical illness, but a primary role. They divide that role into two components: the conscious self-regulation of normally autonomous physiological functions and the interaction of consciousness with biological systems in the body.

What's Offered

A $30 membership fee will entitle you to their two publications, *Artifex* and *Archaeus*, as well as admission to their meetings and use of their extensive library.

Several congresses, which bring together the research of members, are held each year. Topics included in past conferences were:

- Psychoneuroimmunology
- Theology and healing
- Dreams and self-regulation
- Laughter as medicine
- Psychology of illness
- Physiological and psychological responses to music.

Association for Research & Enlightenment, Inc.
P.O. Box 595
Virginia Beach, VA 23451
804-428-3588

Background

Edgar Cayce, America's foremost mystic of this century, lived in Virginia Beach, Virginia, more than 35 years ago. While in a sleep-like state he successfully diagnosed physical ailments and often prescribed remedies that helped alleviate and cure symptoms. Thousands of these "readings"—what he said while in this trance—were transcribed as he spoke.

The Association for Research & Enlightenment (ARE), Inc. explores the implications of his work and disseminates the information found in the more than 14,000 readings.

What's Offered

The $30 membership includes the bimonthly *Venture Inward*, featuring articles on holistic health, meditation, and topics covered in the readings of Cayce. You will also receive monthly articles on one of Cayce's readings and special health reports on his remedies entitled *Holistic Health Research Report*, which details information on one of several hundred specific ailments or health problems.

You may also borrow from the over 400 circulating files of Cayce's readings that include many health topics such as:

- Arthritis
- Allergies
- Tinnitus
- Hypertension
- Obesity
- Migraine headaches.

Members may also borrow information on many of the readings from the Association's library, attend its sponsored conferences, and obtain referrals to physicians who are also members.

When you ask for information you will also receive an extensive catalogue of books, audio tapes, and videos on Cayce and many other health topics.

Australian Wellbeing
P.O. Box 249
Mosman Junction
NSW 2088
Australia

Background

From Down Under comes a full-color, beautifully illustrated bi-monthly ($42 Australian) magazine, *Australian Wellbeing*, touting across its masthead that it will tell you "how to get more out of life."

What's Offered

Arriving every other month, this beautiful magazine presents a bounty of information on health ideas, life experiences, and health and environmental news. Written by both a knowledgeable editorial staff and experts in their field, every story is a good read. Practical rather than theoretical, factual rather than fanciful, each issue will delight as well as inform. From this mélange, a recent issue contained stories on:

- Positive benefits of meditation
- Drugs—risks of even the most commonplace
- Natural immunity boosters—food and herbs
- Weight-loss diets and exercise
- Plant communication
- Medical astrology
- Thai methodology to defeat drug addiction
- Burnout.

Brain/Mind Bulletin
Interface Press
P.O. Box 42211
4717 North Figueroa Street
Los Angeles, CA 90042
213-223-2500

▋ Background

It has been said that understanding the nature of consciousness is the ultimate goal of human knowledge. If so, scientists, philosophers, and researchers are certainly giving it much play.

While predominantly New Age, the monthly ($30) *Brain/Mind Bulletin*, newly renamed the *New Sense Bulletin*, may be a quick and painless way of keeping up with current research in the field.

▌What's Offered

This eight-page newsletter presents summaries of recent research and thinking on both the software of consciousness, the mind, and its hardware, the brain. Each issue consists of 8 to 10 short articles that serve as summaries of a topic in the news. They are scholarly without being pedantic and usually have references for further follow-up. Special features include book reviews and readers' letters. Occasionally, an entire issue is devoted to a single topic such as Ilya Prigogine's chaos theory or new theories about the nature of reality. Examples of topics from recent issues are:

- Right-hemisphere language
- EEG and healing
- Glutamate receptors and DNA
- Seasonal affective disorder and twilight
- Hormone injections and hypertension relief
- Coffee and stress.

You may also purchase back issues and theme packs (bundled articles on a special topic such as learning and creativity, right- and left-brain functions, medicine, psychology and growth, and consciousness and mind). Several guides and audio tapes are also offered.

Center for Frontier Sciences
Temple University
Ritter Hall 003-00   Room 478
Philadelphia, PA 19122
215-787-8487
215-787-5553 (fax)

Contact: Nancy Kolenda, Coordinator

Background

The sheer quantity of new scientific information is staggering, it is estimated that the amount of new information doubles every 10 years. The same can be said of information in alternative healing and the effect of the mind on the body.

The Center for Frontier Sciences (CFS) was established to coordinate and exchange information and to act as a database of resources on information that is on the frontier of science, technology, and medicine.

What's Offered

Affiliation with the Center is reserved for professional researchers and scientists. However, anyone may subscribe to their 30-odd-page quarterly ($25), *Frontier Perspectives*. It includes articles, book reviews, letters to the editor on past articles, a list of upcoming meetings of various groups, and new periodicals. Recent article topics have included:

- Biological effects of low-level radiation
- Homeopathic research
- Bioelectromagnetics
- Regenerative healing in humans
- Unconventional claims in science
- Health promotion through connectedness.

In addition to its newsletter, the CFS hosts round-table discussions at Temple University, many of which are available on audio tape. Recent topics have included:

- Experiments in mind–matter interactions
- Coherence in biology
- Fields and living systems
- Matter and consciousness
- Contrasting views of AIDS etiology
- Consciousness and causality.

Consciousness Village
International Training Center for Rebirthing
and Spiritual Purification
1 Campbell Hot Springs Road
P.O. Box 234
Sierraville, CA 96126
916-994-3737

▌ Background

What is the one thing that we all do without being aware of it? Breathe. Western science and medicine considers breathing an automatic and relatively unimportant matter.

But outside that discipline, breathing is looked upon by many others as an effective means of healing both the body and the mind. Indian, Chinese, and most Oriental medical disciplines believe that proper breathing is an important part in maintaining health and well-being.

In simplified terms, the conscious control of breath is said to increase one's physical energy, and to act as a means of psychological cleansing and balancing.

▌ What's Offered

The conscious control of breathing—establishing specific patterns and relationships between inhalation and exhalation—is taught at Consciousness Village. Besides the training in breathing, the Center publishes a national directory of conscious-breathing teachers.

Institute for the Advancement of Health
16 East 53rd Street
New York, NY 10022
212-832-8282

▌ Background

The Institute for the Advancement of Health (IAH) focuses on the connection between mind and body in both illness and health. The concern is to help the public and health care professionals stay on top of the developing knowledge in the mind-body connection and distinguish fact from fiction, science from hope. Its stated purposes are:

- ▌ To present knowledge of the mind–body health relationship and its treatment in disease
- ▌ To encourage a better patient–doctor relationship.

▌ What's Offered

It is widely (although not universally) accepted that the mind affects the body in everything from headaches to the immune system. Mind–body research has led to many professional intervention treatments: relaxation techniques, biofeedback, meditation, hypnosis, physical exercise, yoga, imagery, and visualization.

A $39 yearly membership entitles you to a subscription to both *Advances* and the *Mind–Body–Health Digest* as well as to attendance at lectures, publication discounts, and access to the Institute's technical staff to discuss other mind-body issues.

The *Digest* (back copies are available free of charge) devotes an entire issue to a topic such as:

- ▌ Cancer, imagery and the immune system
- ▌ Surgery—how the mind affects recovery
- ▌ AIDS—imagery techniques
- ▌ Relaxation and meditation benefits

∎ Arthritis—how the mind affects its pain
∎ Mind–body fitness.

Advances ($10 each for back issues), a technical, scientific journal, has covered topics in greater depth:

∎ Emotions and cancer
∎ Imagery techniques and results
∎ Chronic fatigue syndrome and relaxation techniques
∎ Hypnotic suggestion
∎ Arthritis therapies
∎ Placebo effect
∎ Belief and biology
∎ Personality and disease.

Institute for the Advancement of Human Behavior
P.O. Box 7226
Stanford, CA 94306
415-851-8411
415-851-0406 (fax)

∎ Background

It is often difficult for professionals to find information about alternative treatments that have been proven clinically effective. One of the reasons conferences, seminars, and workshops are held is to remedy that problem. Participants and attendees not only exchange information, but network to continue their studies.

The purpose of the Institute for the Advancement of Human Behavior (IAHB) is to hold conferences on different clinical approaches to emotional problems.

▐ What's Offered

Although for professionals, and not exclusively offering alternative therapies, the IAHB's programs are often at the cutting edge and include much that is called alternative. Examples of topics discussed at recent conferences are:

- ▐ Imagination and healing
- ▐ Laughter and play
- ▐ Treatment of depressive disorders and anxiety
- ▐ Therapies for controlling anger.

Conferences are open to anyone, and audio tapes of past meetings are available.

Institute for the Study of Human Knowledge
P.O. Box 1062
Cambridge, MA 02238
800-222-ISHK

▐ Background

The Institute for the Study of Human Knowledge believes that your mood can affect your body and the treatment you receive for an ailment. Examples are many: Certain fragrances can reduce stress and blood pressure; laughing raises pain thresholds, boosts immunity, and protects against stress; looking at a wooded scene rather than a brick wall from a hospital bed, means going home a day earlier.

▐ What's Offered

The Institute conducts seminars and sells books on the subject of mood medicine. Recent seminars focused on healthy pleasures and:

- Why pleasure and positive moods are critical to psychological and physical health
- How psychological states affect immunity
- Mobilizing positive beliefs
- Mind–body therapies
- Seasonal affective depression treatments
- Eclectic techniques from cognitive therapy, relaxation training, and behavior modification.

An assortment of books and pamphlets written for the lay individual rather than for the professional is also available.

Institute of Noetic Sciences
475 Gate Five Road
Suite 300
Sausalito, CA 94965-0909
415-331-5350

∎ Background

Two Nobel Prize winners—one in physics, the other in chemistry—have said that the most significant Nobel Prize in the year 2000 will be "for the study of human consciousness." The Institute of Noetic Sciences' purpose is to conduct its own research and report on the research of others in the nature and potential of the human mind.

Founded by astronaut Edgar Mitchell, the Institute's research on alternative health involves:

- The mind's influence on physical states of the body
- Communication between the nervous and the immune systems
- Effect of brain behavior and psychological stress on the immune system
- Autoimmunity

∎ Relaxation therapy, biofeedback, hypnosis, exercise, and imaging.

∎ What's Offered

Your $35 membership includes all three Institute publications and its extensive, wide-ranging catalogue of books, reports, audio tapes, and videos.

Its premier journal, the quarterly, *Noetic Sciences Review*, discusses up-to-date concepts in consciousness research, the mind-body connection, and healing. Recent topics have included:

∎ Biology and fighting
∎ Energy medicine
∎ Creative altruism
∎ Emotional exploration
∎ Commitment.

The *Noetic Sciences Bulletin*, a second quarterly members receive, reports on continuing Institute research projects, members' activities in local discussion groups, upcoming conferences, workshops, lectures, and courses.

International Forum on New Science
1304 South College Avenue
Fort Collins, CO 80524
303-491-5753

Contact: Dr. Maury L. Albertson

∎ Background

It is often found that people pushing at the edge of human knowledge see far beyond it. New science in the areas of health range from the alternative healing systems of therapeutic touch, color therapy, electromagnetic healing, and vibrational medicine to the nonphysical dimensions of out-of-body experience, channeling, crystal energy, and near-death experiences.

The International Forum on New Science (IFNS) seeks to bring together much of the information on this new science by providing a forum where these topics may be introduced, discussed, and implemented by both professionals and laypersons.

▌ What's Offered

The IFNS holds conferences and discussions on new science, and publishes original scholarly papers on any new science topic.

While not directly advocating specific alternative therapies to prevent or treat an ailment or disease, if you wish to learn more of what goes on at the edge of alternative healing, you could do worse than contact this new group for more information.

International Institute for Bioenergetic Analysis
144 East 36th Street
New York, NY 10016
212-532-7742

▌ Background

No one is ever completely still; even breathing involves movement. The way we move can be as much a part of personality as speech.

The International Institute for Bioenergetic Analysis (IIBA) believes that the body and its energy processes are a way of understanding personality. The energy processes consist of respiration, metabolism, and movement. The amount of energy you have will determine how you respond to life. This is like the mind–body connection in reverse. The body affects the mind; how you think affects how you feel.

▌What's Offered

Through national affiliate groups and at its headquarters, the IIBA offers several workshops on bioenergetic analysis for the layperson.

A variety of books and monographs are also published on movement and energy and how they relate to personality, feeling, thinking, aggression, stress, illness, and self-expression.

A yearly ($8) journal, *Clinical Journal of Bioenergetic Analysis*, presents articles by the Institute's members.

John F. Kennedy University
12 Altarinda Road
Orinda, CA 94563
415-253-2211

▌Background

Not only are there now once unheard-of health and medical subjects, but new names dress up traditional ones. What once were the questions of Philosophy 101, are now the province of the John F. Kennedy Graduate School for the Study of Human Consciousness.

▌What's Offered

This graduate school offers advanced degrees in a variety of areas of human experience. The two that relate to alternative health care are the masters degree in transpersonal psychology and holistic health.

If you are interested in exploring a career in alternative health or just want to expand your knowledge in a formal classroom, write for a catalogue of degree and nondegree courses.

Meditation
17211 Orozco Street
Granada Hills, CA 91344-1132
800-266-6624
818-360-2059 (fax)

Background

Used by many civilizations throught the ages, meditation is touted for both its health and spiritual benefits.

Meditators seek self-awareness through their relationship to their internal environment and awareness of their relationship to their external environment. Meditation helps in that quest by allowing the individual to stand apart from his or her emotional self through a relaxed body state and a quiet mind.

Meditation, a four-color, bimonthly ($17.95) magazine, has as its stated purpose is to "explore and promote meditation as a consciousness-expanding activity."

What's Offered

Each issue's dozen or so articles fall under the headings of spirituality, education, psychology, science, health/healing, meditation, alternative science, profiles, and interviews. Regular features include letters to the editor and product, music, book, video, and audio tape reviews. All articles are written by acknowledged experts in their fields and each covers its topic well: Background material, quoted material, and practical advice are included. Some recent topics have been:

- Visual meditation
- Codependency and neurolinguistic programming
- Violence and the inner self
- Tantra sexuality
- Photoreading—new learning techniques
- Role expectations—men's psychological health

- Cooking with herbs
- John Bradshaw on psychological healing and the 12-step recovery method
- Rupert Sheldrake on physics and collective intelligence.

National Institute for the Clinical Application of Behavioral Medicine

P.O. Box 523
Mansfield Center, CT 06250
203-429-2238
203-429-7949 (fax)

Contact: Christine Huda, Executive Director

▌Background

The National Institute for the Clinical Application of Behavioral Medicine, an organization for professional health care practitioners, holds conferences for physicians and researchers and reports on clinical findings from around the world.

▌What's Offered

The information presented at a few of their recent conferences has included such topics as:

- Mind and medicine
- Role of consciousness in health
- Healing rituals
- Role of imagery in medicine
- Mind and cancer
- Psychology of health, immunity, and disease
- Psychoneuroimmunology and the mind–body connection

■ Exercise for cardiac patients
■ Negative emotions and disease
■ Biofeedback guided imagery
■ Psychology of immunity.

Audio tapes, videos, workbooks, and written proceedings of all the conferences are normally available.

New Frontier
New Frontier Education Society
46 North Front Street
Philadelphia, PA 19106
215-627-5683
215-440-9945 (fax)

■ Background

However one may view the New Age, much of its emphasis on health is very old-fashioned: diet, exercise, personal responsibility, and self-reliance.

New Frontier, a monthly ($18) calling itself the Magazine of Transformation, is much in the New Age vein.

■ What's Offered

Rather than many different authors in each issue, *New Frontier* has a stable of columnists writing on the same general subject each month. Each month Gary Null writes on alternative health, and Phillip Lansky, M.D., writes on new health findings and their relation to the inner self. Several columns on food and various psychological aspects of health have rotating columnists. All the articles are short—no more than a page or two—and offer practical advice rather than theoretical knowledge. Subjects are covered from an eclectic view rather than toeing a party line. Some recent subjects are:

- New American diet
- Living foods
- Health and laughter
- Environmental medicine
- Barley—preparation and recipes
- Past-life regression therapy
- Verbalization for psychological health
- New Age gourmet cooking
- Dangers of particleboard in construction.

Nurse Healers—Professional Association, Inc.
175 Fifth Avenue
Suite 2755
New York, NY 10010
518-325-3583

▌ Background

Touch—the laying on of hands. This ancient healing art may be the oldest. In Western culture, it is vividly described in the Bible. In Eastern cultures, instructions in its use are found in ancient books of healing.

In the early 1970s, Dolores Krieger, a nurse, and Dora Kunz, a teacher of meditation, developed Therapeutic Touch (TT) to make the practice more scientific and to enable health care practitioners to be trained in its use.

Nurse Healers—Professional Association, Inc., founded by them, trains and certifies professional nurses in the practice of TT.

▌ What's Offered

Touch therapy is said to release the body's accumulated and congested energy. A practitioner will first calm herself through a form of meditation. Then, the client's "energy field" is analyzed through questioning and a kind of sweeping hand and arm movement around the client's body. Finally, the bottled-up energy is released. A touch therapist is said to move the client's energy from points where it is strongest to points where it is weak.

In this very personal form of healing, unlike all of orthodox medicine and most other forms of alternative therapies, the state of mind of the person giving the treatment is considered as important as that of the person receiving the treatment. A practitioner who is angry, sick, or just tired, may obstruct rather than encourage, healing.

The benefits claimed for TT are:

- Anxiety reduction
- Pain relief
- Speeding the recovery of bodily injuries and many diseases.

If you believe that touch therapy is something worth looking into for yourself, write or telephone Nurse Healers for further information on TT and a referral to a practitioner in your area.

Whole Health Institute
4817 North County Road 29
Loveland, CO 80538
303-679-4306

Contact: Kathy J. Basset, Administrator

▊ Background

There are many magazines and journals on alternative health care. There are many organizations of health care professionals and lay individuals who are interested in alternative health care. But seldom does one find a combination of the two.

The Whole Health Institute (WHI) is an organization of professionals and interested individuals seeking to promote a wholistic approach to health and health care. More interested in the causes of health than the cures of diseases, the Institute holds conferences, publishes books and a journal, and sees itself as an educational rather than a medical organization.

▌ What's Offered

A nonprofessional membership ($20) in WHI will entitle you to receive their 24-page quarterly, *Healing Currents*. Its articles are all written by members and almost always deal with an educational and practical approach rather than a theoretical and explanatory one. In other words the information is more concerned with health than with health care. Recent article topics are:

- Spirituality and healing
- Holistic nursing
- Placebo response—efficacy
- Depression—wholistic approach
- Nervous system healing
- Homeostasis—the body's balance point
- Vibrational healing
- AIDS—viral infection or lifestyle disease
- Menopause—self-help diet.

The Institute holds an annual conference open to all professionals and the lay public and publishes several short books and videos on health.

Referrals to health care professionals who are members of the Institute are also available.

Further Resources
   see all resources under IMAGERY
   Balance
   Health Consciousness
   International Society for the Study of Subtle Energies and Energy
      Medicine
   Lifespan Associates
   Sounds True Catalogue
   Spectrum

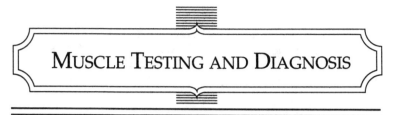

MUSCLE TESTING AND DIAGNOSIS

Biokinesiology Institute
5432 Highway 227
Trail, OR 97541
503-878-2080

Contact: Lynn Vice, Director

▮ Background

A widely used means to test the body's functioning is biokinesiology. A close cousin to applied kinesiology, biokinesiology uses a more simplified approach to muscle tesing and yields specific results.

Basically, here's how muscle testing works. Pressure is applied to a muscle or muscle group. If it responds with normal strength, it is assumed that the muscle is receiving proper nerve stimulation. If it responds with less-than-normal strength, it is assumed that there is an interference with normal nervous system functioning.

This is all tied together because specific organs are linked with specific muscles through the pathways in the neuronal pools of the central nervous system. By testing a specific muscle's strength, you are learning about a specific organ's functioning. When an organ is found to be malfunctioning or functioning below its optimum level, treatment can then be given.

▌ What's Offered

The Biokinesiology Institute offers information on how you can apply biokinesiology yourself. Through the use of group and individual lessons and a variety of books and other material, you will be able to learn the basic principles of biokinesiology and how to apply them.

For those wishing an evaluation by a professional, the Institute maintains a referral list of qualified specialists.

Institute of Behavioral Kinesiology
P.O. Drawer 37
Valley Cottage, NY 10989
914-353-2664

Contact: John Diamond

▌ Background

Behavioral kinesiology is a method of physically testing the body's responses to applied force to evaluate the factors that influence health. It is often combined with an anlysis of emotions called life-energy analysis.

The Institute of Behavioral Kinesiology offers all the books, newsletters, audio tapes, videos, and written materials of Dr. John Diamond, one of the originators of behavioral kinesiology, life-energy analysis, and a new approach to life called cantillation.

▌ What's Offered

The offered material includes information on a variety of topics, some of it far removed from kinesiology. In fact, much of the writing will appear more metaphysical than physical. Nevertheless, some topics from the now defunct newsletter's back issues will give you a better idea of what you can expect:

- Facial expressions and emotions
- Dental applications of behavioral kinesiology
- Doctor–patient relationship
- The thymus in body monitoring
- Stressful TV ads
- Holistic approach to stop smoking
- Fear of the new
- Finding scapegoats
- Deviousness.

As unusual as all this sounds, as far away from alternative health care as it seems to be, much of it has proved beneficial to people in the United States, England, Germany, New Zealand, and Australia.

International College of Applied Kinesiology
P.O. Box 25276
Shawnee Mission, KS 66225-5276
913-648-2828
913-648-2041 (fax)

▌ Background

Applied kinesiology, originally discovered by Dr. George Goodheart almost 30 years ago, has been newly "discovered" by many alternative health care advocates and is now their new mantra. Applied kinesiology is a form of manual muscle testing. The testing is used to evaluate the body's functioning through the movement of the musculoskeletal system. Particular muscles and muscle groups are correlated to different parts of the body.

For example, a weakness in the sartorius muscle indicates a problem in the adrenal gland. Additionally, there are several osteopathic, body reflex points that can be stimulated to the weak part of the body. The concept is similar in theory to that of acupuncture: there are certain points on the body that correspond to organs of the body and stimulating these points helps cure ailments relating to and in those organs.

The International College of Applied Kinesiology (ICAK) is a professional organization and training center for applied kinesiology. Its members include health care professionals who use applied kinesiology in their practice. These normally include physicians, chiropractors, and other manipulative therapists.

▌ What's Offered

ICAK publishes a small number of pamphlets on applied kinesiology along with its bimonthly ($10) newsletter, *Health Capsules*, which contains news of upcoming events, information about new courses, and reviews of scientific literature.

More important to you as a health care consumer, ICAK will provide you with a list of its members in your area from which a practitioner can be selected.

Touch For Health Foundation
1174 North Lake Avenue
Pasadena, CA 91104-3797
818-794-1181

∎ Background

Touch involves more than intimacy or violence. It can be used to diagnose ailments and body imbalances.

Touch For Health (TFH) uses touch for "muscle-testing." The Foundation's muscle testing method, like others such as applied kinesiology, enables someone to determine a body's energy flows and levels. This information can be used for allergy and food testing, left/right brain integration, and maximizing athletic performance by:

- Increasing energy and improving muscle strength and flexibility
- Strengthening the immune system and speeding up healing time
- Reducing stress and depression
- Relieving sprains, headaches, and low back pain.

∎ What's Offered

Touch For Health conducts classes in a system that integrates acupuncture and massage therapy. Courses may be taken by anyone interested in learning the technique for themselves.

TFH membership ($30) includes a subscription to their bimonthly newsletter, *Touch For Health*. Its features include a calendar of upcoming classes and special events, developments in the field from readers, and new techniques and applications.

A membership directory is available from which you can find a qualified and trained practitioner in your area.

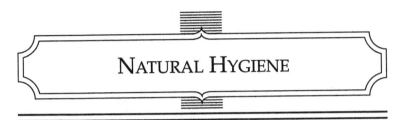

NATURAL HYGIENE

American Natural Hygiene Society
P.O. Box 30630
Tampa, FL 33630
813-855-6607

▋ Background

Natural hygiene is a vegetarian health regimen emphasizing raw foods, such as vegetables, nuts, and seeds, and food combining; eating foods in a certain order to help their assimilation in the body.

The American Natural Hygiene Society (ANHS) is a professional organization promoting the benefits of natural hygiene to the general public.

▋ What's Offered

A $25 membership fee entitles you to the ANHS magazine, *Health Science,* which has articles on nutrition, fasting, and self-care, recipes, interviews with natural hygiene authorities, and readers' queries.

Several conferences and seminars for members are held throughout the year, and audio tapes and books are available.

A professional referral list is available for those wishing to consult a natural hygienist in their area.

Bionomics Health Research Institute
P.O. Box 36107
Tucson, AZ 85740
602-297-0798

▌ Background

Quite possibly the oldest systematic American theory of health and disease, scientific articles, journals, and books on natural hygiene date back more than 150 years.

The Bionomics Health Research Institute (BHRI) publishes and distributes a variety of material on natural hygiene.

▌ What's Offered

BHRI's material is published in a series of four courses or books. The two courses on applied nutrition cover food combining, vitamins, minerals, enzymes, cooked foods, metabolism, weight gain and loss, and health cookery. The lifestyle management course discusses natural hygiene as an integral part of life and periodic fasting. The course on pathology discusses both common and chronic ailments, exercise, health, and beauty. The material is well researched, up-to-date in its material and health findings, and purposefully written for the lay individual.

An eight-page newsletter, *Health-O-Gram*, is published 10 times a year ($13.50). In it you will find several articles on health and prevention from a natural hygiene viewpoint and a recipe or two. Most issues have reprints of articles written by famous health and medical authorities of the past. For example, a recent issue discussed the Koch germ theory.

International Association of Professional Natural Hygienists
204 Stambaugh Building
Youngstown, OH 44503
216-746-5000
Contact: Mark A. Huberman

▌ Background

Natural hygiene, aside from the nutritional benefits of strict vegetarianism as a means of disease prevention and wellness, stresses the importance of supervised periodic fasting.

The International Association of Professional Natural Hygienists (IAPNH) is a professional organization of legally licensed medical doctors, osteopaths, chiropractors, and naturopaths who practice natural hygiene in their own lives and use it in their professional practice.

▌ What's Offered

IAPNH's quarterly newsletter ($12) is available to nonmembers. The articles are concerned with the professional practices of supervised fasting, case studies, book reviews, and members' letters.

Referrals to practitioners in your area are also available when you write or telephone.

Life Science Institute
1108 Regal Row
P.O. Box 609
Manchaca, TX 78652-0609
512-280-5566

▌ Background

The Life Science Institute provides an extensive array of information on a health discipline called "life science," a form of natural hygiene. Aside from its philosophical bent against most of the orthodox medical profession and its emphasis on self-help, life science believes in a strict form of vegetarianism consisting of eating mostly raw foods and proper food combining.

The raw foods are made up primarily of fruits, vegetables, nuts, and seeds. A few cooked foods are permitted, but only in moderation. Food combining emphasizes the need to eat only certain foods together and in a certain order. This practice is said to aid digestion and stimulate the complete absorption of nutrients.

▌ What's Offered

A multilesson, home-study course as well as audio tapes are available on life science, the nutrition and health practices advocated by the Institute. Part of the course material are two newsletters: *The Healthway Advisor* responds to readers' questions with health advice, and *The Health Science Newsletter* comments on and discusses the current health scene. Both are published monthly.

An additional bimonthly magazine ($18), *Healthful Living*, is also published. It too stresses natural hygiene and its importance in maintaining good health. Recent topics of information discussed have included:

- Medical health care—negative appraisal
- Arthritis—relief through diet
- AIDS—immune system revitalization
- Food combining—enhancement of utilization and bioavailability
- Recipes
- Stretching exercises.

Also sold are a wide variety of food preparation and health products, audio tapes, videos, and books. Topics in this material are natural hygiene, gardening, recipes, pregnancy, and natural child care.

Natural Hygiene, Inc.
P.O. Box 2132
Huntington Station
Shelton, CT 06484
203-929-1557

▌ Background

The word *hygiene*, from the Greek, refers to health. Natural hygiene is certainly a philosophy and probably a science that studies and applies the conditions (it finds) upon which life and health depend.

Natural Hygiene, Inc. is an educational institute disseminating information on natural hygiene and how it applies to health today.

▌ What's Offered

A $15 membership entitles you to the 26-page bimonthly, *Journal of Natural Hygiene,* a pocket-sized magazine of health articles written by professional health care practitioners who apply natural hygiene in their practice. Each article gives practical advice for the problem it discusses. A few recent topics that have been discussed are:

- ▌ Problems with prescription drugs
- ▌ Calcification and acid-forming foods
- ▌ Water-logged tissues
- ▌ Natural dental care
- ▌ Nontoxic pest control
- ▌ Fear as a killer.

Aside from a catalogue of natural hygiene books, audio tapes and videos, a custom research service on over 700 health topics is also available.

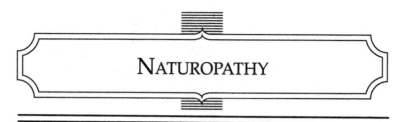

NATUROPATHY

American Association Of Naturopathic Physicians
Suite 200
2800 East Madison Street
Seattle, WA 98112
206-323-7610

Contact: John Weeks, Executive Director

▌ Background

The American Association of Naturopathic Physicians is the professional association for naturopathic medical practitioners. They will send interested individuals general information on naturopathic medicine and maintain a national directory of naturopathic physicians (N.D.s).

▌ What's Offered

An N.D. has a Doctor of Naturopathic Medicine degree from a four- or five-year graduate-level naturopathic medical college. Where licensed and regulated, N.D.s must pass a national or state-level examination.

Naturopaths are trained as specialists in the use of natural therapeutics and are primarily concerned with restoring overall health rather than alleviating symptoms. An N.D. performs physical examinations, laboratory tests, gynecological examinations, nutrition and dietary assessments, metabolic analysis, allergy tests, and other diagnostic tests and performs minor surgery.

Among the therapies of naturopaths are:

- Clinical nutrition—nutrition and the therapeutic use of foods
- Botanical medicine—the use of plants as medicinal agents
- Homeopathy—highly diluted preparations used to strengthen the body's immune responses
- Physical medicine—manipulation of muscles, bones, and spine
- Counseling and stress management
- Oriental medicine—acupuncture, acupressure, and oriental botanical medicine
- Natural childbirth—prenatal and postnatal care.

A telephone call will get answers to questions about naturopathic medicine and a referral to a practitioner in your area.

Journal of Naturopathic Medicine
The Journal Management Group, Inc.
10 Morgan Avenue
Norwalk, CT 06851
203-661-7375

▌ Background

Naturopathy, unfortunately, remains relatively unknown to most people. It is looked upon as folk wisdom by many orthodox physicians. Yet, modern naturopaths use the same scientific principles to prescribe their treatments.

Until recently, most information about naturopathy was available only in lay publications and textbooks from naturopathic colleges. Other rigorous naturopathic information was available to the professional through seminars, workshops, and conventions.

The quarterly ($65) *Journal of Naturopathic Medicine* publishes articles on original research and clinical studies that use naturopathic treatments.

▌ What's Offered

Far too expensive and technical for the nonprofessional, the journal will prove of benefit to any health care professional seeking rigorous, scientific information on more holistic treatments for common and chronic ailments.

All the articles conform to the same standards one expects from professionally oriented scientific journals: background, patient studies, data, treatment methods, and extensive references. Regular features include literature and book reviews, legislative news, letters to the editor, and research abstracts. Topics discussed include:

- Colonic irrigation—serum electrolyte effect
- Endocrine functioning—inhibition through botanical agents
- Mood-altering ketosis—dietary factors in carbohydrate-restricted diets
- Nutrition—prevention and treatment of neoplasia
- Hodgkin's lymphoma.

Further Resources
Homeopathic Academy of Naturopathic Physicians
Lafayette University

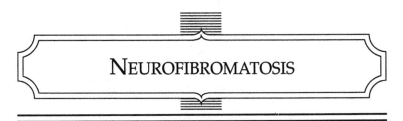

NEUROFIBROMATOSIS

National Neurofibromatosis Foundation, Inc.
141 Fifth Avenue
Suite 7-S
New York, NY 10010
800-323-7938
212-460-8980 (NY state)
212-529-6094 (fax)

Contact: Kim Robinson

∎ Backgound

Neurofibromatosis (NF) is a group of genetic disorders that make tumors grow along certain nerves. It is inherited from a parent with NF or caused by a spontaneous mutation in the sperm or egg cell. NF affects one out of every 4000 individuals, usually in early childhood. There is no cure for NF. No one has yet discovered the genetic mechanism for its onset.

The National Neurofibromatosis Foundation (NNF), Inc., and its 22 local chapters provide psychological help and genetic and educational counseling to persons with NF and their families. Their long-range mission is:

- ∎ To promote and support research
- ∎ To provide information and assistance to sufferers of NF
- ∎ To act as an NF resource for health care professionals.

▌ What's Offered

A single information package with more than enough material for you to learn about NF is sent on request. NNF also sells several technical monographs, children's books, and videos.

Their eight-page, quarterly ($25), *neuro*fibroma*tosis*, will keep you informed about the organization and what's happening in NF research. Recent issues have discussed:

- ▮ Optic glioma
- ▮ Gene mapping
- ▮ Local chapter news
- ▮ Research findings.

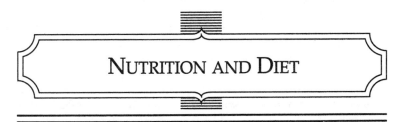

NUTRITION AND DIET

American Board of Nutrition
9650 Rockville Pike
Bethesda, MD 20814
301-530-7110

▌ Background

Most professionals—lawyers, accountants, and physicians to name just three—are required to have certain educational requirements and to pass examinations attesting to their competence.

The American Board of Nutrition (ABN) helps establish standards in the field of human or clinical nutrition and certifies those who pass the examinations. Analogous to medical specialty boards, persons who meet the ABN's qualifications are called diplomates in human or clinical nutrition. Certificates in "Clinical Nutrition Specialist" are given to M.D.s. Ph.D.s receive certificates in "Human Nutrition Specialist."

▌ What's Offered

If you believe such certification important in choosing a health care professional, the ABN will supply you with a list of qualified professionals in your state who are in private practice. Your request should include a self-addressed, stamped envelope.

American College of Nutrition
722 Robert E. Lee Drive
Wilmington, NC 28412-0927
919-452-1222

▌ Background

The American College of Nutrition conducts classes, holds meetings, conducts conferences and seminars, and generally promotes nutritional education for physicians, researchers, and medical school students.

▌ What's Offered

While only professionals may join, the College also publishes the *Journal for the American College of Nutrition* every other month and a quarterly newsletter. The journal serves as a means of disseminating basic and clinical nutrition information and relevant findings in the field of medical nutrition. It is technical and is definitely not for the layperson with only a casual interest. Some topics covered in recent articles have included:

- Malnutrition in infant and adult diseases
- Nutrition and cancer
- Nutrition and cardiovascular disease
- Nutrition and hypertension
- Disease modification through nutrition.

The newsletter is less technical, covering clinical nutritional news in a jargon-free style.

A telephone call or letter will get a technical question on nutrition answered. With some persistence you can get through to one of the College's expert staff, all of whom are physicians.

American Institute of Nutrition
9650 Rockville Pike
Bethesda, MD 20814
301-530-7050

■ **Background**

The American Institute of Nutrition (AIN) is the principle professional organization of nutrition research scientists in the United States. It acts as a networking facilitator to promote interaction among nutrition researchers throughout the world.

■ **What's Offered**

Membership is not open to the layperson. However, the AIN publishes the prestigious *Journal of Nutrition*, devoted solely to nutritional research. It also includes peer-reviewed experimental research findings, critical reviews of new findings, and commentaries on a wide range of nutrition topics.

You will find the journal at every college or university library offering degrees in the biological or health sciences. It is worth inspection for those having more than a casual interest in the field.

American Journal of Clinical Nutrition
American Society for Clinical Nutrition, Inc.
P.O. Box 64025
Bethesda, MD 21201
301-571-8303

■ **Background**

Nutrition can be thought of as the body's utilization of nutrients. Thinking that every nutrient in what you eat or drink is used in some way is just plain wrong. Digestive disorders, poor food combining, a lack of enough stomach acid, and a host of other maladies can contribute to little or even no benefit to much of the food you eat and the liquids you drink.

The American Society for Clinical Nutrition (ASCN), Inc., the professional organization of clinical nutritionists in medicine and the health sciences engaged in research and teaching in colleges and universities, publishes the *American Journal of Clinical Nutrition* ($70).

▌ What's Offered

Although membership in the ASCN is not open to the lay public, anyone may subscribe to the journal. This peer-reviewed journal is considered by many to be the premier journal in the field of nutrition. It often contains breakthrough discussions years before the medical profession or the popular media ever hears of it.

American Nutrimedical Association
P.O. Box 25113
Colorado Springs, CO 80936
719-591-2659

▌ Background

Nutrimedicine is the medicine of diet, nutrition, and disease prevention. Health then, must be the responsibility of the individual. The health care practitioner is a guide offering advice and education as well as treatment. Specifically, that entails:

■ Influences of polluted air and impure water
■ Detoxification of the body
■ Impact of overwork and lack of exercise
■ Relationship between stress and illness
■ Effect of negative thoughts and feelings.

The American Nutrimedical Association (ANA) is a professional organization of licensed nutritional counselors.

■ What's Offered

Membership in ANA is open only to licensed practitioners who may also be chiropractors, naturopaths, dieticians, or nutritionists.
A membership directory is published every year and may be used to find a professional in your area.

American Nutritionists' Association
5530 Wisconsin Avenue, NW
Suite 1149
Washington, DC 20815
301-657-4751
301-656-0989 (fax)

■ Background

Many people believe that a dietician is the same as a nutritionist. Not so. A dietician primarily learns about food preparation and food service for an institution such as a hospital. A nutritionist has a degree, often an advanced one, in human nutrition science or a related health field such as biochemistry or public health.
Wouldn't you like the choice to pick a nutritionist or dietician as you think best? Well, you can't in Montana, North Dakota, or

Tennessee. Many states have already enacted laws that preclude anyone other than a member of the American Dieticians Association from practicing nutrition—or even speaking on nutrition and diet. This practice is likely to grow.

The American Nutritionists' Association (ANA) is a professional organization of nutritionists, most of whom have advanced degrees. It focuses on the twin goals of further education and political advocacy against the exclusion of nondieticians from practicing nutritional counseling.

▌ What's Offered

ANA publishes *The Nutrition Report*, an eight-page monthly newsletter ($50) highlighting the latest in nutritional news and research results.

If you are seeking a qualified nutritionist to assist you in your health goals, finding one affiliated with the ANA will assure you of his or her abilities.

American Vegan Society
501 Old Harding Highway
Malaga, NJ 08328
609-694-2887

▌ Background

It is no longer a secret that the American diet of high fat, high cholesterol, high protein, low fiber, and low carbohydrates contributes significantly to the high incidence of heart disease, diabetes, circulatory illness, some cancers, and many other serious health problems that plague us.

The American Vegan Society advocates a strict vegetarian diet of no meat, fish, fowl, eggs, dairy, or honey on ethical as well as on health grounds.

∎ What's Offered

The Society's quarterly ($18), *Ahimsa*, features discussions on every aspect of vegetarianism, all from health, ethical, and environmental viewpoints. They also sell several unusual vegetarian cookbooks, publications, audio tapes, and videos.

Hippocrates Health Institute
1443 Palmdale Court
West Palm Beach, FL 33411
407-471-8876

∎ Background

By now everyone has heard that sprouts are good for you; many people add them to their lunch salads. Some people know of the health benefits of vegetable and wheatgrass juices; a few of them make fresh vegetable or wheatgrass juice every morning.

Much of the research into these rich sources of enzymes, vitamins, and minerals began with the Hippocrates Health Institute.

∎ What's Offered

For $25 you will receive a subscription to their triannual, *Hippocrates Newsletter*; a copy of the book *The Hippocrates Health Program*, and a catalogue of wheatgrass juicers, food dehydrators, water purification systems, enzymes, and algae for you to prepare your own enzyme-rich juices. Each newsletter issue includes recipes, an editorial, and a variety of short articles on such topics as:

- Science of breathing properly
- Benefits of the placebo effect
- Eating live foods
- Aftereffects of cesarean deliveries
- Lawn chemicals
- Nontoxic homemade cleaners
- Fluoride dangers
- Colonic irrigation.

International Journal of Biosocial and Medical Research
Life Sciences Press
P.O. Box 1174
Tacoma, WA 98401
206-922-0442

▌Background

The *International Journal of Biosocial and Medical Research*, coming out twice a year ($25), publishes original studies and their findings on behavior and its relation to nutrition, neurotoxicology, and environmental health.

▌What's Offered

This publication is not for the faint of heart. The writing is scientifically rigorous and not free from technical terms and jargon. But, the scientific findings will not be found anywhere else for years. Topics covered in the past few issues are:

- Freshwater sources of omega-3 fatty acids

- Spontaneous regression of cancer
- Decaffeinated beverages and female fertility
- Nonseasonal depression
- Alcoholism and nutritional therapy
- Aluminum and Alzheimer's disease
- Full-spectrum lighting to overcome depression.

Back issues are available, along with several original books on subjects that are not to be found anywhere else, including work on:

- Blood pH and diet
- Zinc treatment of eating disorders
- Diet and crime.

Natural Healing Newsletter
FC&A Publishing
103 Clover Green
Peachtree City, GA 30269
404-487-6307

▌ Background

Natural Healing Newsletter, an eight-page newsletter of one- and two-page articles from scientific journals, provides the reader with news from both the medical and natural health fields.

▌ What's Offered

Articles run the gamut from natural health to medicine-related problems to practical preventive advice. Much of the information is taken from respected medical and health journals from around the world or reported in major general-interest publications or newspapers. Each issue contains up to two dozen articles on a wide variety of topics. Most articles have references for follow-up study. The short quarter-page summaries always include practical advice on implementing the health-related suggestions. Topics covered from several recent issues are:

- Dangers of too little dietary cholesterol
- Bone cancer—links to fluoride
- Chemotherapy and leukemia
- Milk and colon cancer
- Sleep and longevity
- Potassium and blood pressure
- Side effects of glaucoma eyedrops
- Alzheimer's disease
- Crash diets and gallstones
- Salt and osteoporosis.

North American Nutrition & Preventive Medicine Foundation, Inc.
1280 West Peachtree Street
Suite 2209
Atlanta, GA 30367
404-876-3060

Contact: Bonnie Jarrett, Director

▌ Background

The North American Nutrition & Preventive Medicine Foundation (NAN&PMF), Inc. provides orthodox physicians, Ph.D.s, and other health care practitioners with information and professional skills to enable them to incorporate preventive medicine. Primarily an educational resource for these professionals, it provides specific treatments, modalities, and concrete information on promising research.

▌ What's Offered

Conference and seminar proceedings are often published in book or audio-cassette form. Both are sold by the Foundation. Recent topics presented at NAN&PMF conferences include:

- Acid/alkaline nutrition balancing—determining your blood's pH
- Homeopathic medicines
- Macro and micro minerals—what the body needs
- Amino acid metabolism—increased bioavailability
- Immunological evaluation
- Cancer chemoprevention—diet and nutrition.

While not its primary objective, referrals to qualified practitioners in your area are also available by writing or telephoning.

North American Vegetarian Society
P.O. Box 72
Dolgeville, NY 13329
518-568-7970

▌ Background

I've already said much about the health benefits of vegetarianism. Others write and speak eloquently of the benefits vegetarianism has on the environment and of the pain and suffering imposed on animals by the slaughter for our food.

The North American Vegetarian Society, a nonprofit, educational organization promoting a vegetarian way of life, addresses all three issues.

▌ What's Offered

Membership ($18) includes a subscription to the Society's quarterly newsletter, *Vegetarian Voice*. The newsletter keeps readers up to date on medical and nutritional studies and offers many unusual vegetarian recipes with well-researched, one- or two-page articles, each with references and citations for follow-up study. Additionally, it provides advice for members to promote vegetarianism among consumers and speaks out on environmental and animal rights issues. Topics discussed from a recent issue were:

- Four vegetarian food groups—wheat grains, vegetables, legumes, and fruit
- Drinking water—are we running out?
- Soy and rice milks—product evaluations
- Fat and calories.

Several vegetarian cookbooks and books on vegetarian nutrition are also available, as well as information on local vegetarian organizations across the country.

Nutrition Action Healthletter
Center for Science in the Public Interest
1501 16th Street, NW
Washington, DC 20036
202-332-9110

∎ Background

Published 10 times a year ($9.95) by the prestigious Center for Science in the Public Interest (CSPI), the 20-page-plus *Nutrition Action Healthletter* will keep you current with information on a variety of health topics gleaned both from many publications and from the Center's own studies. Some of the information is so new that you may wind up knowing more than many professionals.

∎ What's Offered

Every issue is divided into six sections: readers' letters, commentaries on health news, health and science topics, special feature articles, eating, and new supermarket items. Article topics have included:

- Pesticide residues in food
- Fat and the diet—how much is too much
- Foods to lower blood pressure
- Eating to reduce cancer risks
- Fish oils—benefits and harm
- Food additives—how they affect health
- Calcium
- Garlic benefits
- Alternatives to fast food.

Your subscription includes a discount to other CSPI publications and two useful nutrition and food posters. The Center is so convinced that you will like the *Nutrition Action Healthletter* that they offer a full refund at any time during your subscription.

The Center also sells many health books and a diet software program as well.

Nutrition Education Association, Inc.
3647 Glen Haven
Houston, TX 77025
713-665-2946

∎ Background

A 1986 National Restaurant Association study concluded that nearly 46 million Americans eat fast food every day of their lives. Yet more people than ever say that they're chronically tired. Many people feel vaguely ill at least a few days every week. Hyperactive children seem to be everywhere, and parents complain that their kids are driving them crazy while children say the same thing about their parents.

Instead of this all being in their heads, it may be in their stomachs; so says Dr. Ruth Long of the Nutrition Education Association, Inc.

∎ What's Offered

Long contends that many of our daily ills—cancer, allergies, heart attacks, high blood pressure, hyperactivity, stress, arthritis, and depression—can be both linked to the typical American diet and prevented or controlled by eating the right foods and taking the proper nutrient supplements.

Aside from her numerous books and articles on nutrition and cancer, the Nutrition Education Association also publishes a 12-lesson home-study course in nutrition. The course contains information on supplemental nutrients and a diet that stresses natural wholesome foods and the elimination of junk foods, coffee, tea, colas, cocoa, canned and bottled drinks, and alcohol.

Nutrition News
P.O. Box 55279
Riverside, CA 92517
714-784-7500

▌ Background

To keep up with what's happening in nutrition would mean spending hours each day reading, which is far too much for anyone other than the devoted professional. However, the interest in nutrition expressed by many has led to many popular magazines, newsletters, journals, and books.

Nutrition News, a monthly ($18), four-page newslettter often distributed in health food stores, is one of them.

▌ What's Offered

Each issue contains a detailed article on a single subject. The one I am now looking at is entitled "Echinacea and Chamomile." The article is thoroughly researched with quotations from many sources. For example, a 1986 German study is cited. Of 203 women with candida albicans, half were given echinacea as part of an ointment; after six months, 84% of the women using echinacea remained free of infection. Several resources are usually given at the end of each article. This issue also had short pieces on preparing your own herbal remedies and on making your own herbal suntan lotion. Past issue topics have included:

- ▌ Osteoporosis—exercise, calcium, estrogen replacement, and diet
- ▌ Blood sugar (hypoglycemia and diabetes)—GTF chromium, l-glutamine, and vanadyl sulphate
- ▌ Colon health—intestinal bacteria
- ▌ Raw glandulars—adrenal, pancreas, thyroid, liver, and brain
- ▌ DLPA and pain control.

Nutrition Report
Health Media of America, Inc.
1873 Playa Riviera
Cardiff, CA 92007
714-784-7500

Background

The monthly ($48) eight-page *Nutrition Report* is written for professional health care practitioners.

What's Offered

For its material, *Nutrition Report* scans more than 8000 scientific journals every month and reports on important research and findings in vitamins, minerals, and other nutrients. Its format is technical but succinct, with the emphasis on the practical rather than the theoretical. Each issue contains one or two guest editorial articles by respected authorities in the health field who look at the latest information on a specific topic and offers guidance for disease treatment or minimum individual nutrient requirements. Other articles, each less than a page long, summarize an important finding or study and draw practical conclusions from it. References accompany articles for further study. Recent topics discussed have included:

- Sugar and disease
- Beta carotene and cancer
- Retinol and lung cancer
- Fish oil and carcinoma
- Vitamin E and epilepsy
- Guar gum and minerals
- Prenatal thiamin deficiency.

While important information is presented, this newsletter is not intended for the average individual looking to extend his or her nutrition knowledge. But, if you are scientifically literate and have a deep desire for the latest in nutrition information, an inquiry will get you a sample copy.

Physician's Committee for Responsible Medicine
P.O. Box 6322
Washington, DC 20015
202-686-2210

▌ Background

In spite of what many people believe, whenever a patient describes his or her symptoms many physicians do not automatically turn to the *Physician's Desk Reference* to find a drug to treat it. Nor does every specialist loom to surgery as the only procedure to treat the diseases in which he or she specializes. Instead, thousands of physicians are turning toward preventive medicine.

The Physician's Committee for Responsible Medicine (PCRM) provides solid, well-grounded, thoroughly researched nutritional information for the general public and other physicians.

▌ What's Offered

The primary source of information from the PCRM is the 16-page, bimonthly ($14.95) *Guide to Healthy Eating*. It contains a completely original feature: tear-out recipes for your own file. Also included are updates on the latest research in food and nutrition in exceptionally well-researched material. Every article contains dozens of scientific references for its conclusions. In other words, this magazine reads like a scientific journal, except that the rest of us can understand and enjoy it. Sample topics recently covered are:

▪ Foods for athletes—gaining a competitive edge

- Vegetarianism—guide for teenagers
- Exotic vegetables—health benefits
- Poultry—dangers
- Vtamin E—immunity.

Joining the PCRM ($20) will entitle you to a subscription to *PCRM Update*, a 12-page, bimonthly newsletter. Its articles on nutrition are more for the health care professional than the lay individual, but the serious student of nutrition and health will find much of value in its articles. Needless to say, it also has many scientific references and gives the lay reader an excellent perspective on just how much of many nutrients are recommended and why.

Preventive Medicine Update
International Academy of Holistic Health & Medicine
218 Avenue B
Redondo Beach, CA 90277
213-540-0564

▌ Background

Preventive medicine, by definition, goes against the grain of establishment medicine. Without the qualifying adjectives and weasel words, preventive medicine says that you are responsible for your own health and what you do can keep you healthy, and establishment medicine says do what you want and when you get sick we will treat you.

The International Academy of Holistic Health & Medicine (IAHHM) is clearly in the prevention camp. Its stated priorities are:

- To educate the public to the importance of good health habits
- To make people aware of the adverse side effects of all drugs and to point to the alternatives that exist

I To work toward nutritional education of dieticians and to establish a nutrition information network
I To emphasize the importance of the environment and health
I To promote freedom of choice in health care.

I What's Offered

Preventive Medicine Update is IAHHM's monthly ($18) publication. Its features include book reviews and a calendar of upcoming events. Articles are written by professionals and present short, thoroughly researched views on recent findings from around the world. A few topics from recent issues are:

I DMG and the immune response in aging
I Magnesium supplements for the heart
I Tumor necrosis factor and cancer
I AIDS and cell therapy.

Send a self-addressed, stamped envelope to the IAHHM for a referral to a preventive doctor in your area as well as a recent issue of their journal.

Price-Pottenger Nutrition Foundation
P.O. Box 2614
La Mesa, CA 92044-2614
619-582-4168

Contact: Chris Castagna, Office Manager

I Background

The Price-Pottenger Nutrition Foundation publishes and distributes a wide variety of books, audio tapes, videos, bibliographies, reprints, and articles on a variety of medical disease-prevention subjects and nutrition as well as the quarterly *Nutrition Journal.*

▎ What's Offered

The motto of the Foundation is: "Our goal is to make nature's simple but profound message of optimum good health available to everyone." With that in mind, here are just a few of the topics for which you can obtain information in the form of pamphlets and reprints:

- Tooth and gum care—prevention through nutrition
- Fish oils—benefits to the heart
- Vitamin E, niacin, and vitamin C as antioxidants
- Herbal medicine
- Nutrition for parents
- Candida albicans—nutritional and dietary guidelines.

Recent article topics from *Nutrition Journal,* a journal devoted to health and disease prevention through nutrition, include:

- Refined sugars—how they affect you
- Gardening and children
- Sprouting—increased nutrients
- Organic food sources—mail-order suppliers
- Understanding food labels.

Solstice
Solstice Magazine, Inc.
310 East Main Street
Suite 105
Charlottesville, VA 22901
804-979-4427

▌ Background

Solstice, a monthly ($36), 34-page magazine of macrobiotics, focuses its attention both on personal and environmental health.

▌ What's Offered

A practical rather than theoretical magazine, *Solstice* has a hands-on, how-to slant in each of its articles and monthly columns; even the readers' letters are serious-minded and eclectic. Regular features include seasonal recipes and a macrobiotic directory. Recent issues have addressed the following topics:

- Vitamin B_{12} shortages in vegetarians
- Water in the home
- Quinoa—a new grain for cooking
- Dowsing to find water
- Organic growing and rock dust
- Hazards of manmade magnetism
- Children's herbs.

Vegetarian Resource Group
P.O. Box 1463
Baltimore, MD 21203
301-366-VEGE

▌ Background

The Vegetarian Resource Group, through its publications, conferences, workshops, and seminars, promotes and encourages vegetarianism.

▌ What's Offered

Vegetarian Journal ($20) is published six times a year and is primarily concerned with giving practical advice for vegetarians such as meal planning, vegetable nutrition, recipes, health aspects of a vegetarian diet, and the economic benefits of vegetarianism. Recent articles have included:

- 28-day meal planner
- Weight-loss guide
- Vegetable sources of calcium to prevent osteoporosis
- Indian recipes
- Egg replacers and dairy substitutes
- Athletics and vegetarianism.

They also sell many unusual vegetarian cookbooks, including kosher ones, and books dealing with the special problems of the elderly and children.

Vegetarian Times
Vegetation Life & Times
P.O. Box 570
Oak Park, IL 60303
708-848-8100
708-848-8175 (fax)

▌ Background

Vegetarian Times is a monthly ($12.47 for six issues) magazine promoting and encouraging vegetarianism.

▌ What's Offered

Vegetarian Times concerns itself primarily with practical advice for vegetarians. That includes meal planning, vegetable nutrition, recipes, health aspects and benefits of a vegetarian diet, and the ecological advantages of vegetarianism. All recipes and food tips are divided into three sections: one for ovolacto (foods that contain eggs and dairy) vegetarians, second for lacto (foods that contain dairy but not eggs) vegetarians, and a third for vegans (foods that contain neither dairy nor eggs) vegetarians. Recent article topics have included:

- Low-fat desserts—no sugars or artifical sweeteners
- Weight-loss guide
- Natural hygiene
- PMS—herbal treatments
- Impotence—how diet can affect it
- Health benefits of vegetarianism
- Chemical-free farming—pesticides
- Vegetarian news.

Vegetarian cookbooks, including ethnic and specialty foods, as well as books dealing with ecology and animal rights are also available by mail.

Further Resources
 see all resources under ORGANIC FOOD
 see all resources under ORTHOMOLECULAR NUTRITION AND
  THERAPY
 American Health Federation
 American Institute for Cancer Research
 Better Nutrition for Today's Living
 Cooking for Survival Consciousness
 Delicious
 Environmental Nutrition
 Foundation for Innovation in Medicine
 Healing Currents
 International Academy of Nutrition and Preventive Medicine
 Let's Live
 Macrobiotics Today
 Natural Health
 Natural Lifestyle and Your Health
 Nutrition and Cancer
 Nutrition for Optimal Health Association, Inc.
 Preventive Medicine Update
 Princeton BioCenter
 Safe Water Foundation
 Today's Living
 Total Health

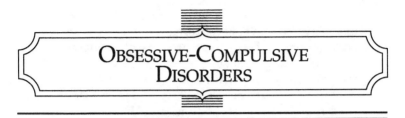

OBSESSIVE-COMPULSIVE DISORDERS

Obsessive Compulsive Information Center
University of Wisconsin Department of Psychiatry
600 Highlan Avenue
Madison, WI 53792
608-263-6171

▌ Background

Every person has habits. Most of us brush our teeth and comb our hair the same way every morning. But if we combed our hair constantly, that habit would become a compulsion. People sufferering from obsessive-compulsive disorders constantly exhibit habitlike behaviors.

The Obsessive Compulsive Information Center was founded by the University of Wisconsin to serve as an information clearinghouse for OCD. Updated every day, more than 4000 references from journals, books, government documents, seminar and meeting procedures, unpublished manuscripts, and reports are entered into a computerized database. Currently, topics referenced include:

- Obsessive-compulsive disorder
- Obsessive-compulsive spectrum disorders
- Obsessive-compulsive personality disorder
- Obsessions
- Compulsions
- Trichotilomania.

▌ What's Offered

The University Center, a nonprofit organization, charges a nominal fee for its computerized printouts that consist of bibliographies and copies of articles. In addition to this service, physician referral and support group lists are also available.

A 62-page booklet (revised in 1991) entitled *Obsessive Compulsive Disorders: A Guide* is published under the University's auspices. It serves as a guide for people with OCD and their families and the general public.

OCD Foundation, Inc.
P.O. Box 9573
New Haven, CT 06535
203-772-0565

Contact: James W. Broach, Executive Director

▌ Background

Obsessive-compulsive disorder (OCD) sufferers have recurring, unwanted, and unpleasant thoughts (this is the obsession part of the ailment) and/or perform ritualistic behaviors that they feel driven to perform (this is the compulsion part).

Obsessions can be about anything: dirt (continually cleaning), fear of acting violently (excessive timidity), concern with order (excessive neatness), inability to discard possessions (never throw out useless or worn-out possessions), or almost anything else. Compulsions run from continuous handwashing, hoarding, acting from obsessional fears, and always touching things over and over.

The OCD Foundation, Inc. is an organization of individuals suffering from OCD, their families, and professionals who treat them. The Foundation's primary concern is with intervention, control, and cure. With this in mind, educational programs, research into causes and therapies, and support to families are provided.

▌ What's Offered

Joining the organization for $25 will bring you further information in the form of several booklets, put you in touch with a local group, and may lead to referrals for professional counseling.

The *OCD Newsletter*, the OCD Foundation's eight-page, bimonthly bulletin, has well-researched articles on various compulsions (most written by acknowledged experts and containing references for further follow-up research), a readers' question column, news of new treatments and therapies, and information about upcoming events. Topics recently covered include:

- ▌ Childhood obsessive-compulsive behaviors
- ▌ Treatment at UCLA
- ▌ Cognitive behavioral therapy
- ▌ Gambling.

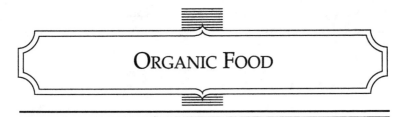

Organic Food

Green Earth
Green Earth Natural Foods
2545 Prairie Street
Evanston, IL 60201
618-864-8949

Contact: Kyra Walsh, Editor

■ Background

Green Earth is a quarterly ($14) 40-page journal devoted to providing information about food and ecology. Since you are (at least to a certain extent) what you eat, what you eat is a matter of how healthy you are.

■ What's Offered

Divided into five sections, this easy-to-read journal presents more than a dozen two- to four-page, well-researched articles—often reprints from other alternative publications—on food, growing food, and personal ecology in each issue. You will also find news tidbits and short pieces on other resoruces. A sample of subjects from recent issues is:

- ■ Pesticides and children's health
- ■ Organic farming
- ■ Raw juice therapy
- ■ Fats and oils from vegetable sources
- ■ Indoor air quality
- ■ Lab-tested produce.

Green Earth Natural Foods is a mail-order, organic food store that offers an extensive array of vegetables and fruits—all organically grown—the year round.

Natural Food and Farming
Natural Food Associates
P.O. Box 210
Atlanta, TX 75551
214-796-3612

▌ Background

Natural Food and Farming, a monthly ($20) magazine, is exclusively devoted to the benefits of organically grown food: eating it and growing it.

▌ What's Offered

Although many articles for organic food growers are included, the primary purpose of *Natural Food and Farming* is to provide readers with information on the benefits of whole foods.

Besides the articles, the magazine has a continuing farmer's market and classified section in which you will find dozens of farms that sell organically grown produce, chickens, and meats directly through the mails. Article topics are evenly divided into health and nutrition, food, and gardening sections. A regular monthly cooking section features a discussion of ethnic cooking along with samples of recipes. Recent topics that nonfarmers would find of interest are:

- Vitamins and whole foods
- Food fallacies
- Biointensive garden pest management

■ Spearmint—cosmetics and cooking
■ Creole cooking.

Organic Network
Eden Acres
12100 Lima Center Road
Clinton, MI 49236-9618
517-456-4288

■ Background

There is a rush to buy organic food. Local health food stores are now as likely to have packaged organically grown food as vitamin supplements and herbal preparations.

But what about organic produce and farmer's markets: fruits and vegetables, as well as meat and poultry (if you are not a vegetarian)? These are often much harder to come by. To fill this void, in steps *Organic Network*.

■ What's Offered

Organic Network is a 2½-inch-thick, three-ring, bound book listing organic farmers, health food stores, organizations, and holistic doctors.

The complete national directory runs $20 and includes the binder. If you just want the listing for your own state, send $2.

Sprout House
40 Railroad Street
Great Barrington, MA 01230
413-528-5200

▌Background

Many people believe that to get the protein they need, they must eat meat. A few who know better believe that their protein must come from legumes, grains, and rice. Both groups are wrong. Normally, low-protein foods increase their protein up to 300% when they're sprouted.

Sprout House sells a variety of seeds suitable for sprouting as well as much nutritional educational material.

▌What's Offered

First and foremost there are sprouts—everything from the adzuki red bean to the yellow soybean. Along with the 30-plus varieties of seeds, Sprout House sells a variety of unusual bamboo and flaxseed sprouters.

A bimonthly ($15) newsletter, covering the nutritional benefits of sprouts, growing techniques, and product reviews always has short, practical articles. An example of topics from a recent issue includes:

- Nutritional values—alfalfa versus iceberg lettuce
- Different kinds of sunflowers
- Sprout nutrition—chromagraph analysis
- Hydrogen peroxide—remove mold and clean fruit and vegetables.

Additionally, there are a number of nutritional books and audio tapes on vegetable growing, juice fasting and detoxification, sprouting, and wheatgrass.

Sproutletter
Sprouting Publications
P.O. Box 62
Ashland, OR 97520-9989
800-543-5888
503-488-2326

▌ Background

Anyone who has had a salad in a restaurant or perused the produce counter at a local supermarket has likely eaten mung bean and alfalfa sprouts and has assumed that since they're in a salad they must be good for us. Unfortunately, too few people know of the nutritional value and health benefits of live, enzyme-rich foods such as sprouts. Too few of us think that only a few seeds can even be sprouted, unaware that many unusual seeds—buckwheat, corn, lentils, lettuce—are among the 39 seeds that can easily be sprouted in the kitchen.

Sproutletter, a quarterly ($10) newsletter, is devoted to teaching you how to sprout, what to sprout, and the health benefits of sprouts as food.

▌ What's Offered

This four-page newsletter's regular features include recipes, book and product reviews, and interviews with live-food experts. All the articles stress only the practical: getting the most from sprouting and eating healthier with sprouted seeds. Article topics from past issues have included:

- Sprouting mucilaginous seeds
- Calorie/protein relationship
- Tryptophan inhibitors
- Spirulina, chlorella, green manna
- Nutrients in germinated seeds
- Sprouted wheat blends

- Riboflavin in wheat
- End of nutrition chain
- Hydroponic sprouting.

If you have even a passing interest in a better diet with a wider variety of foods, sample back issues are available for $2.50 and may be worth your scanning.

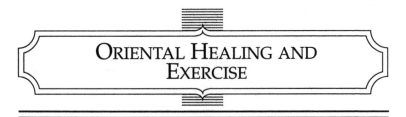

ORIENTAL HEALING AND EXERCISE

Acupressure Institute of America
1533 Shattuck Avenue
Berkeley, CA 94709
800-442-2232
415-845-1059

▌ Background

Traditional acupressure relieves muscular tension by stimulating traditional acupuncture points on the body with touch. Acupressure is said to release tension and repressed emotions and to increase body awareness.

The Acupressure Institute of America (AIA) offers certified training for professionals in Oriental bodywork for:

- ▌ Arthritis relief
- ▌ Sports acupressure
- ▌ Emotional balancing
- ▌ Traditional Oriental therapy
- ▌ Stress management
- ▌ Women's health.

▌ What's Offered

The AIA offers many audio tapes and workbooks for self-acupressure and relaxation techniques.

A practitioner referral service to a qualified, professional, traditional acupressurist is also available if you telephone or write.

American Academy of Medical Acupuncture
5820 Wilshire Boulevard
Suite 500
Los Angeles, CA 90036
213-937-5514
213-937-0959 (fax)

▌ Background

Only recently has acupuncture begun to be used by medical doctors. In fact, one form of acupuncture is practiced only by physicians who have been trained in acupuncture as a specialty. Medical acupuncture is used to promote health and well-being, to prevent illness, and to treat various medical conditions. Some of these conditions are digestive disorders; respiratory disorders; neurological and muscle disorders; and urinary, menstrual, and reproductive problems.

The American Academy of Medical Acupuncture (AAMA) was founded by physicians who use medical acupuncture as part of their practice.

▌ What's Offered

Aside from treatment, the AAMA offers training to physicians who wish to incorporate acupuncture into their professional practice.

When requested, the AAMA also provides referrals to qualified physician acupuncturists in any area of the country.

American Foundation of Traditional Chinese Medicine
1280 Columbus Avenue
Suite 302
San Francisco, CA 94133
415-776-0502

Contact: Barbara Locke

▮ Background

Traditional Chinese medicine, despite the popularity of acupuncture and Oriental herbal preparations, is still relatively unknown in the United States.

That successful treatments exist for migraine headaches, arthritis, diabetes, gynecological problems, skin problems, asthma, and many other chronic and degenerative conditions finds Western allopathic medicine skeptical. Nonetheless, some therapies have proven themselves successful for thousands of years.

The American Foundation of Traditional Chinese Medicine (AFTCM) believes that a synthesis of the two disciplines—allopathic and Oriental—can offer more than either medical system alone. To that end it not only uses and encourages the use of Eastern therapies in clinics and hospitals, but also encourages scientific research of the entire body of traditional Chinese medicine.

▮ What's Offered

Some of AFTCM's projects include teaching Chinese medicine to health care professionals and holding classes for the general public. It also publishes an eight-page, quarterly newsletter, *Gateways*, that contains case studies, book reviews, and clinical information on the uses of acupuncture, herbs, moxibustion, and qi gong (therapeutic breathing exercises).

AFTCM also maintains an international referral network of traditional Chinese medicine practitioners and can refer you to one in your area.

Center for Traditional Acupuncture
American City Building
Suite 108
Columbia, MD 21044
301-997-3770
301-596-6006 (hotline)

▌ Background

More people have been treated with Chinese medical treatments throughout history than any other system of medicine. Part of this natural system is acupuncture: a system of inserting special needles just beneath the skin's surface at special points or meridians on the body. Acupuncture has been used successfully for treating a wide range of ailments such as headaches, allergies, chronic fatigue syndrome, depression, back pain, digestive disorders, joint pain, menstrual disorders, infertility, sleeping problems, asthma, addictions, and stress.

The Center for Traditional Acupuncture is one of the nation's leading exponents of the Chinese system of acupuncture.

▌ What's Offered

Aside from acupuncture treatment at its clinic, the Center offers certified clinical training leading to a masters degree. Seminars for the public on Chinese healing are conducted on a regular basis and include:

- Expanding the view of health and illness
- Chinese philosophy of healing
- Taking charge of your own wellness.

An extensive catalogue of materials on natural healing methods, acupuncture for the layperson and the professional, and Oriental philosophy is available.

A telephone call to their hotline will get you a referral to a qualified, traditional acupuncturist in your area.

G-Jo Institute
P.O. Box 8060
Hollywood, FL 33084
305-791-1562

▌ Background

Everyone of us is subject to minor bodily ailments and aches and pains: burns, muscle aches, night leg cramps, low back pain, and headaches. Most of us shrug it off. A few take a drug from the local pharmacy. Some visit the doctor for stronger relief.

Many cultures cannot afford these luxuries. Oriental cultures use various forms of self-help, among them acupuncture and acupressure.

▌ What's Offered

The purpose of the G-Jo Institute is the dissemination of information to the general public about self-help, "self-health" techniques to be used as alternatives to over-the-counter drugs. All the techniques were designed to be used by anyone. The method used is a simple, three-stage, acupressure process to relieve pain and other minor ailments.

The G-Jo Institute has a large catalogue consisting of over a dozen books, audio tapes, and videos.

When you write or telephone for your catalogue it will likely be accompanied by a small folder entitled *Self-Health Report*, a foldout of the basics of G-Jo with several illustrations on how it works for a few minor ailments. Try the technique yourself; a pleasant surprise may await you.

Internal Arts Magazine
P.O. Box 1777
Arlington, TX 76004-1777
800-223-6984
817-860-0129
817-460-5125 (fax)

▌ Background

Many of the Chinese exercise disciplines, qi gong, baguazhang, and tai jiquan among them, are said to promote physical health and emotional well-being, especially related to those maladies associated with stress and environmental factors.

These claims have been confirmed by tests conducted at the Beijing Institute of Traditional Medicine. Based upon alpha and beta brain-wave activity reduction, taijiquan has been shown to reduce stress. Achievement of target heart rate and reductions in percentage of body fat were attained using baguazhang.

▌ What's Offered

Internal Arts Magazine, a bimonthly ($18.95), devotes much of each issue to qi research and development from both traditional and scientific perspectives. Written by the world's leading authorities in the internal martial arts fields, articles are fact-filled and thoroughly researched. Most articles are practical and help the practitioner develop his or her skills. Regular features include:

- Qi gong
- Baguazhang
- Taijiquan
- Meditation
- Herbology
- I Ching
- Aikido.

Internal Arts Magazine also has an extensive catalogue of books and videos on Eastern exercise disciplines and philosophies.

International Foundation of Oriental Medicine
42-62 Kissena Boulevard
Flushing, NY 11355
718-321-8642

▌ Background

What appears to be new and startling to Western medicine is old hat to Oriental medicine. Acupuncture continues to find new adherents and practitioners as it is seen to provide relief to many ailments.

The International Foundation of Oriental Medicine (IFOM) is a professional organization of health care practitioners encouraging research, setting standards of practice, and exchanging information about new uses for and new modalities of acupuncture.

▌ What's Offered

What is of major benefit to you as a health care consumer is the Foundation's national registry of members.

If you write or telephone, the IFOM will answer your questions about acupuncture and refer you to a qualified, licensed, and trained acupuncturist or physician in your area who uses acupuncture.

International Institute of Reflexology
5650 First Avenue North
P.O. Box 12642
St. Petersburg, FL 33733-2642
813-348-4811
813-381-2807 (fax)

▌ Background

Reflexology employs a constant pressure on points (called reflexes) in the feet that correspond to each of the organs in the body through the 72,000 nerve endings found on both the top and bottom of the human foot. Stimulating the reflexes properly is supposed to help many health problems. Its use is primarily to relax tension and improve nerve and blood supply.

The International Institute of Reflexology (IIR) teaches practitioners-to-be the Ingham method of foot and hand reflexology.

▌ What's Offered

The IIR sells books and visual aids to enable anyone to practice reflexology on himself or herself successfully.

For the consumer, who may also attend some of the introductory seminars, the IIR also provides referrals to qualified reflexologists.

International School of Shiatsu
22-28 South Main Street
Doylestown, PA 18901
215-340-9918

∎ Background

Shiatsu, one of the many manipulative therapies, uses firm pressure on various parts of the skin called pressure points. This massage-related discipline is designed:

- ∎ To balance the body
- ∎ To relieve tension
- ∎ To bring pain and muscle-fatigue relief
- ∎ To reduce strees.

The International School of Shiatsu (ISS) is an accredited school for training professionals and is recognized by many massage therapy professional organizations.

∎ What's Offered

ISS gives lectures, professional training, and courses for the interested individual in:

- ∎ Shiatsu
- ∎ Muscle testing
- ∎ Muscle balancing
- ∎ Bodywork
- ∎ Body–mind mechanics
- ∎ Massage therapy.

The school will also provide referrals to qualified and certified shiatsu practitioners in your area.

Jin Shin Do Foundation for Bodymind Acupressure
366 California Avenue
Suite 16
Palo Alto, CA 94306
415-328-1811

▌ Background

Almost everyone has heard of acupressure to relieve either chronic or transient pain. What many people do not know is that there are many kinds of acupressure.

What makes the jin shin do system so different from other acupressure methods is its use of different pressure points. So unique is this approach that the Jin Shin Do (JSD) Foundation for Bodymind Acupressure's advanced classes are taken by physicians, physiologists, and psychotherapists.

▌ What's Offered

Although a professional organization offering state-certified courses, the JSD Foundation also sells many books, audio tapes, videos, and reports including ones that will teach you how to use Jin Shin Do acupressure on yourself or a family member.

The JSD Foundation will also refer you to a professionally trained acupressurist in your area.

National Commission for the Certification of Acupuncturists
1424 16th Street, NW
Suite 105
Washington, DC 20036
202-232-1404

Contact: Karen E. Wilson

▌ Background

It is often quite difficult to judge the qualifications of a professional. Doctors and lawyers display their diplomas in their offices and are licensed.

But what of acupuncturists? Seventeen states independently license them. Eleven allow acupuncturists to practice only under supervision. Eighteen restrict the practice to physicians. Four have entirely different rules.

The purpose of the National Commission for the Certification of Acupuncturists (NCCA) is to rectify that and bring national certification to the practice of acupuncture. And they seem to be succeeding: More than half the states licensing acupuncturists have already adopted their certification examination.

▌ What's Offered

For the health care consumer who desires that his or her acupuncturist be certified by a nationally recognized group, the NCCA's directory of members is offered for sale.

National Council of Acupuncture Schools and Colleges
P.O. Box 954
Columbia, MD 21044
301-997-4888

▌ Background

Acupuncture in America hasn't the long tradition of medicine and established medical schools. If there's a Johns Hopkins University or Cornell Medical University of acupuncture, I'll bet few people would recognize its name.

The National Council of Acupuncture Schools and Colleges (NCASC) serves as a national accreditation council to evaluate residential schools and colleges of acupuncture and Oriental medicine. It helps:

- ▪ To develop faculty programs to improve teaching
- ▪ To provide guidance for membership school programs
- ▪ To support member schools toward their accreditation.

▌ What's Offered

NCASC will send you a list of schools that it has accredited. You may then telephone or write to any one of the colleges to ask questions: general questions about acupuncture, the kind of acupuncture specialty you may need for a particular condition or ailment, or a list of their graduates who are currently in practice in your area.

Shen Systems
221 East Market Street
Suite 304
Iowa City, IA 52245
800-432-5846

▌ Background

Oriental medicine is far more than acupuncture, herbal mixtures, and strange-looking exercises. Many of these teachings—perhaps the most important of them—still remain relatively unknown in the West. Among them is qi gong, a method to channel and circulate your inner energy through acupuncture meridians.

▌ What's Offered

Shen System offers a series of videos from the First International Training Course for Medical Qi Gong Practitioners, held in 1988 just outside of Beijing. The tapes are taught by five Oriental qi gong masters and dubbed in English.

T'ai Chi
Wayfarer Publications
P.O. Box 26156
Los Angeles, CA 90026
213-665-7773

▌ Background

T'ai chi, sometimes called Chinese yoga, is an ancient Chinese discipline of health that includes the practices of relaxation, meditation, self-defense, and self-cultivation.

▌ What's Offered

T'ai Chi, published six times a year ($20), provides information about all the aspects of the discipline that are said to have reputed health benefits in healing hypertension, gastric problems, arthritis, heart disease, and anemia. The stretching exercises and meditation are said to improve circulation, help relax and strengthen the nervous system, and reduce stress. Issues include articles on the physical and psychological aspects of this philosophical approach to better health.

Wayfarer, its parent company, also sells a variety of books and videos on t'ai chi and qi gong (another of the Chinese disciplines of health).

Yoga Journal
2054 University Avenue
Suite 604
Berkeley, CA 94704-1082
415-841-9200

▌ Background

Yoga is more than a series of strange-looking exercises. Rather, it also encompasses holistic healing, psychology, bodywork and massage, martial arts, and meditation. The yoga techniques for breathing and body positioning are designed to improve mental as well as physical agility and to reduce tension.

The 120-page, bimonthly ($12) *Yoga Journal* focuses on body–mind techniques to personal, physical, and spiritual health.

▌ What's Offered

Yoga Journal's colorful articles are written by leading yoga and environmental authorities and stress practical application rather than theory and philosophy. A regular feature includes an extensive review of books, audio tapes, and videos. Recent topics that have been dealt with are:

- ▌ Bitter herbs and health
- ▌ Chinese healing
- ▌ Preventing osteoporosis—exercise, diet, and yoga
- ▌ Addictions.

Further Resources
Health World

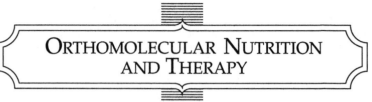

ORTHOMOLECULAR NUTRITION AND THERAPY

Canadian Schizophrenia Foundation
7375 Kingsway
Burnaby
British Columbia, Canada V3N 3B5
604-521-1728

▌ Background

Schizophrenia, according to the Canadian Schizophrenia Foundation, is not a split personalty. Rather, it is a group of biochemical diseases that affect personality—changing the way a person sees, hears, tastes, thinks, and feels. Its treatment is a nutritional one known as orthomolecular psychiatry.

The Canadian Schizophrenia Foundation, much like the Huxley Institute for Biosocial Research, believes that not only can schizophrenia be helped, but that it may be preventable. Their information program includes:

- ▌ A publication list of more than 200 books, pamphlets, and article reprints
- ▌ Publication of the *Journal of Orthomolecular Medicine* ($30) for health professionals
- ▌ Publication of *Health and Nutrition Update* for laypersons focusing on brain ailments
- ▌ Conducting conferences on nutritional medicine.

What's Offered

Your annual ($25) membership fee will entitle you to receive the quarterly, *Health and Nutrition Update*. Aside from articles on biosocial studies, cookbook reviews and diet, general orthomolecular topics, nutritional medicine, vitamin and mineral supplementation, trace elements, and mineral analysis, it has well-researched articles written by clinicians and scientists on natural therapies for:

- Alcohol and drug abuse
- Allergies, sensitivities, and ecological illness
- Candida albicans
- Cardiac and immune system illnesses such as cancer and AIDS
- Hypoglycemia help through diet and supplementation
- Mental disorders, including depression, Alzheimer's disease, Down syndrome, and stress
- Schizophrenia.

The *Journal of Orthomolecular Medicine* may be ordered directly by writing or telephoning their editorial offices at:

16 Florence Avenue
North York
Ontario, Canada M2N 1E9
416-733-2117
416-733-2352 (fax)

Huxley Institute for Biosocial Research, Inc.
900 North Federal Highway
Boca Raton, FL 33432
800-783-3801
407-393-6167

Contact: Mary E. Haggerty, Director

▌ Background

The Huxley Institute for Biosocial Research, Inc. publishes and
distributes a wide variety of books, audio tapes, and articles on
many medical and disease-prevention subjects as well as the quarterly newsletter, *Getting Better*, and the *Journal of Orthomolecular
Medicine*.

▌ What's Offered

Your yearly membership ($25) includes a directory of hundreds of
holistic health care professionals throughout the United States and
a year's subscription to *Getting Better*. Recent issues have included
articles on:

- Tourette's syndrome—what it is and how it can be treated
  using nontoxic methods
- Vitamin D—how the body utilizes it
- Autism—nontoxic therapies
- Drug abuse—nutrient treatments
- Caffeine—the harm it can do
- Attention-deficit disorders in children—what can be done
  with diet and vitamin megadose therapy.

Pamphlets, booklets, and audio tapes on a wide variety of
health-related matters and many ailments are sold for modest
amounts. Included are:

- Depression—megavitamin therapy
- Anxiety and stress—its relation to nutrition
- Immune system disorders—nutritional deficiencies
- Cancer—alternative treatments
- Childhood disorders
- Allergies—testing and treatment with diet
- Cardiovascular disease prevention.

The quarterly ($100) *Journal of Orthomolecular Medicine,* published for professionals, includes studies, reports, and case histories such as:

- Orthomolecular medicine in preventive medicine
- Nutrition and behavior disorders
- New discoveries in minerals and trace elements
- Orthomolecular psychiatry
- Advances in Alzheimer's disease
- Nutrients to age without senility.

Princeton BioCenter
862 Route 518
Skillman, NJ 08558
609-924-8607

Background

The Princeton BioCenter, although primarily an outpatient clinic, is also a research center. Its primary areas of concern involve essential nutrients, trace metal levels, essential fatty acids, the nutritional aspects of schizophrenia, and many aspects of orthomolecular approaches to medical treatment.

■ What's Offered

Aside from its clinical practice in southern New Jersey, the Center has an extensive list of low-priced publications. Topics include:

- Nutrition and mental illness—orthomolecular approach
- Mental illness—elemental nutrients
- Thinking disorders—biochemical immunology
- Vitamin B6—psychiatric case studies
- Birth defects—zinc, manganese, chromium, and vitamin deficiencies
- Hypoglycemia—nutritional answers
- Food allergies—self-diagnosis
- Molybdenum supplementation—biochemical effects
- Drinking water—toxic metals
- Copper—excessive amounts and disease
- Prostaglandins—brown fat and weight loss.

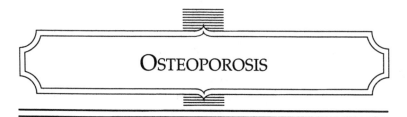

OSTEOPOROSIS

National Osteoporosis Foundation
2100 M Street, NW
Washington, DC 20037
800-621-1773
202-223-2226
202-223-2237 (fax)

Contact: Sandra C. Raymond, Executive Director

▮ Background

Our bones make up the inner structure of our bodies. As long as they are strong, we can stand, sit, move. But if they are weakened—fragile and brittle—our bodies cannot remain strong and healthy.

More than 24 million Americans—almost all of them women—suffer from a condition that makes the bones more and more porous as they grow older. The condition is known as osteoporosis. So debilitating is this condition that an activity as ordinary as bending over to pick up a book can cause bone fractures.

The National Osteoporosis Foundation (NOF) was founded to provide up-to-date information on osteoporosis to patients, health care professionals, and interested individuals. NOF's goals are:

- ▪ To provide support for research
- ▪ To seek to increase public awareness and knowledge about osteoporosis
- ▪ To educate physicians and other health care professionals on the latest scientific information and therapies
- ▪ To inform patients and their families about osteoporosis and the treatments available.

∎ What's Offered

Membership ($25) in NOF includes a subscription to the Foundation's quarterly, *The Osteoporosis Report*, a helpful booklet on prevention and care and periodical news on new medical breakthroughs. The quarterly presents information on upcoming meetings and conferences, research reports, events, clinical updates, and special feature articles on prevention and care.

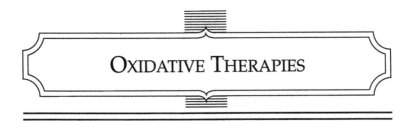

OXIDATIVE THERAPIES

ECH2O2, Inc.
P.O. Box 126
Delano, MN 55328
612-972-2144

Contact: Walter O. Grotz

Background

Many of us have hydrogen peroxide in our bathrooms and know it as a topical disinfectant. What most people don't know is that it is currently being used internally as a therapeutic agent for many ailments.

ECH2O2's purpose is to provide information about the therapeutic benefits of hydrogen peroxide.

What's Offered

For $3 you will get a basic information packet consisting of a report on oxygen therapy and a sample copy of the *ECHO Newsletter*. The *ECHO*, a 20-page, triannual ($10 for two years), is devoted to reporting on the medical uses of hydrogen peroxide. Many reports and booklets on the variety of uses for oxidative therapy are available.

Those of you with vegetable gardens might be interested in the numerous reports of increased growth and improved quality with hydrogen-peroxide–based feed.

International Association for Oxygen Therapy
P.O. Box 1360
Priest River, IA 83856
208-448-2504

▌ Background

Oxygen, the stuff of life, may also be the bane of disease. It is an undisputed fact that many harmful bacteria and disease germs cannot live in an aerobic or oxygen-rich medium; they require an anaerobic or oxygen-poor medium to thrive. Logic would suggest—along with several Nobel Prize winning scientists—that enriching the body with oxygen would be a medical treatment for disease. So it was in America; so it is now in many areas of the world.

The purpose of the International Association for Oxygen Therapy is to promote the reacceptance of various oxygen therapies through public education and training of professionals in its use.

▌ What's Offered

If you have an interest in the health benefits of oxidation therapy, this organization has an extensive collection of information that it makes available. A $25 membership fee gets you a subscription to their newsletter, a list of the reports they have prepared, and details about several oxidative treatments such as:

- ▌ Oxygen therapy blass
- ▌ Ozone therapy
- ▌ Koch therapy
- ▌ Pau d'arco, taheebo, and ipe roxo teas
- ▌ Mucorhicin.

International Bio-Oxidative Medicine Foundation
P.O. Box 61767
Dallas/Fort Worth, TX 75261
817-481-9772

Contact: Edward Baker, Jr.

▌ Background

Oxidative therapy—in this case, the intravenous injection of very weak solutions of hydrogen peroxide—is used to encourage healthy oxidation in cells and tissues. It has shown considerable success in the treatment of:

- ▌ Heart and blood vessel diseases
- ▌ Pulmonary diseases
- ▌ Infectious diseases
- ▌ Immune disorders
- ▌ Miscellaneous ailments such as parkinsonism, Alzheimer's disease, migraines, chronic pain, and certain cancers.

The International Bio-Oxidative Medicine Foundation is a scientific and educational organization formed to promote the use of oxidative therapies.

▌ What's Offered

The $30 annual membership includes a subscription to the quarterly newsletter intended to keep the layperson informed of progress in oxidative therapies. Recent articles have discussed the usage of hydrogen peroxide in AIDS and HIV-positive patients, malignancy, chronic fatigue syndrome, environmentally sensitive individuals, soft tissue healing, asthma, and peripheral vascular disease.

Reprints of articles and the proceedings of past conferences and the *Journal of Bio-Oxidative Therapy* may also be purchased.

A referral to a qualified physician in your area who uses bio-oxidative therapy as part of his or her treatment may also be obtained.

Further Resources
Foundation for Research of Natural Therapies

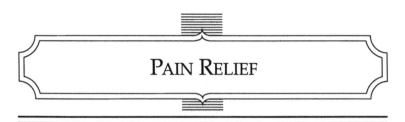

PAIN RELIEF

American Academy of Osteopathy
1127 Mount Vernon Road
P.O. Box 750
Newark, OH 43055
614-366-7911

▌ Background

Osteopathy advocates the theory that body structure and function are totally interdependent. Thus, if the body's structure is altered, the function immediately alters as well. The converse is also believed to be true: A functional alteration causes an immediate structural one.

Osteopathic physicians, although licensed to prescribe drugs and perform surgery, use manipulative techniques to relieve pain and muscular tension on the musculoskeletal system and advise patients on nutrition and exercise to assist the healing process. So popular is osteopathy that a recent survey found that 25 million Americans prefer a Doctor of Osteopathy to M.D.s.

The primary objectives of the American Academy of Osteopathy (AAO), a professional organization of osteopathic physicians, are:

▐ To develop diagnostic techniques and training programs in osteopathy
▐ To analyze the successful methods used and develop means of training other professionals in them.

▌ What's Offered

The primary publication of the AAO is the *AAO Journal*. This 28-page magazine focuses on manipulative techniques, business matters relating to the profession, and news of upcoming events, seminars, and workshops.

Of primary interest to medical consumers is that the AAO will help you find a D.O. in your area.

American Association of Orthopaedic Medicine
5147 Lewiston Road
Lewiston, NY 14092-1956
716-284-5777
716-688-9633 (fax)

▌ Background

Back pain, whiplash, and sports-related injuries are common ailments that seem as different as chalk from cheese. But their commonality is that they are all disorders of the musculoskeletal system.

Dedicated to improving the standards of diagnosing and treating musculoskeletal disorders, the American Association of Orthopaedic Medicine (AAOM) is a professional organization of physicians, dentists, and physiotherapists. AAOM's primary aims are:

- To advance the standards of orthopaedic medicine
- To promote professional training and education
- To stimulate research.

▌ What's Offered

AAOM publishes a journal and a newsletter and conducts several workshops throughout the country.

More to the purposes of the health care consumer, the AAOM will help you locate a member in your area where orthopaedic therapy is advisable.

American Chiropractic Association
1701 Clarendon Boulevard
Arlington, VA 22209
703-276-8800

▌ Background

There are more than 10½ million chiropractic patients and close to 50,000 chiropractors in the United States. Chiropractic doctors, relying on the body's inherent and natural recuperative powers, practice a branch of physiological therapy relating to spinal biomechanics and musculoskeletal, neurological, and vascular problems.

Chiropractors believe that the correction and rebalancing of the spine (called subluxation) will normalize the body's associated nerve, muscle, and vascular disturbances. Briefly, chiropractic modalities include:

- Structural adjustments—correct and rebalance the spine or pelvic bones to relieve nerve, muscle, and vascular disturbances
- Dietary and nutrition—recommend vitamin and mineral supplements to prevent the onset or to lessen the degree of severity of nervous system dysfunctions
- Supportive measures—use of supportive devices and braces to guard against reinjury and to assist healing.

The American Chiropractic Association (ACA) is a professional organization and accrediting agency of chiropractic physicians.

▌ What's Offered

The ACA will send you material on:

- What chiropractic is
- How to choose a chiropractor
- The educational requirements necessary to be a chiropractor
- How to know if you need a chiropractor.

The ACA will also answer any questions about chiropractic care and provide you with information about products that may affect your physical health and spine (such as mattresses, chairs, and pillows).

American Massage Therapy Association
1130 West North Shore Avenue
Chicago, IL 60626
312-761-AMTA

▌ Background

Massage does more than make you feel better. It can, when applied by a skilled professional, contribute signicantly to health and well-being, especially for the relief of pain and to reduce stress. There are seven broad areas of massage therapy:

- Swedish massage is used to improve circulation and relax muscle tension
- Deep-muscle connective tissue massage relaxes chronic tension
- Trigger-point therapy (myotherapy) relieves pain and diminishes muscle spasms
- Shiatsu and acupressure are used to release blocked energy and to increase energy flow

- Reflexology has similar results to shiatsu and acupressure
- Polarity therapy attempts to harmonize the body's energy flow and structural balance
- Hydrotherapy is used as an adjunct to massage and includes hot packs and ice applications along with saunas, steam baths, and whirlpools.

The American Massage Therapy Association (AMTA) is a professional organization and accrediting agency for massage therapists.

▌ What's Offered:

AMTA offers certification programs to graduates of approved schools and publishes two quarterlies, *Massage Therapy Journal* and *Hands On*.

Part of AMTA's stated goals are to provide access to massage therapists. If a massage therapist is a member of AMTA, you may be sure that he or she has successfully completed an approved educational curriculum and meets minimum standards of competency.

AMTA also maintains a national referral service should you wish to find a massage therapist in your area.

American Naprapathic Association
5913 West Montrose Avenue
Chicago, IL 60634
312-685-6020
312-282-2686

▌ Background

Naprapathy is a manipulative therapy, like Feldenkrais or Hellerwork or Alexander technique. It is based upon the premise that the body can heal and restore itself when its biochemical and structural components are in balance. Thus, naprapathy includes nutrition as well as manipulation as treatment.

While stressing prevention, treatment consists of posture and ligament adjustment for injury, shock, physical distortion, and stress. A diet based upon vegetarianism is recommended for biochemical imbalance.

The American Naprapathic Association coordinates its activities with the Chicago National College of Naprapathy and publishes the *Voice of Naprapathy*.

▌ What's Offered

A telephone call or letter will get you several pamphlets and a copy of the *Voice*. In the packet you'll find an explanation of naprapathic medical practices, and several brochures on headache, tension, and bursitis. The *Voice* is a 12-page, 5-by-8-inch journal, with articles written by naprapathic doctors for other practitioners and interested individuals. In many issues you will find articles on:

- ▌ Diet
- ▌ Case histories
- ▌ Treatment modalities
- ▌ Brief overviews of medicine and health.

A written request or telephone call will also get you a referral to a naprapath in your area.

American Osteopathic Association
142 East Ontario Street
Chicago, IL 60611-2864
800-621-1773
312-280-5861

▌ Background

Osteopathy is based upon two underlying principles:

■ The musculoskeletal system is the central component of body; manipulation of that system provides for diagnosis and treatment

■ The body has a natural inclination toward health and to resist disease—preventive medicine, nutrition, and keeping fit can assist in the healing process.

Doctors of Osteopathy (D.O.) are licensed physicians able to prescribe drugs and perform surgery as well as practice osteopathic medicine. The American Osteopathic Association (AOA) is a professional organization of osteopathic physicians.

■ What's Offered

The AOA will provide you with a referral to a D.O. or accredited osteopathic hospital in your area and will direct you to one of the 15 colleges providing osteopathic education.

Associated Professional Massage Therapists & Bodyworkers
1746 Cole Boulevard
Suite 225
Golden, CO 80401-3210
303-674-8478
303-674-0859 (fax)

■ Background

Anyone who has had a professional massage swears by it. Aches, pains, muscle and joint stiffness subside, and an entirely relaxed feeling results.

The Associated Professional Massage Therapists (APMT) & Bodyworkers is a professional organization of massage therapists.

▌ What's Offered

Membership, a subscription to their quarterly newsletter, and continuing education are only available to professional massage therapists or students.

However, the APMT maintains a national referral list and will direct you to one of its members in your area.

Aston-Patterning
P.O. Box 3568
Incline Village, NV 89450
702-831-8228

▌ Background

We are all creatures of physical habit. These habits create physical patterns. How we sit, stand, and move are all done in the same way day after day. These ways are the patterns our body has developed over time. Patterns are often developed to compensate for discomfort, an injury, or a person's immediate environment. These patterns can often accumulate stress and tension in certain areas of the body.

Aston-Patterning conducts a series of training courses for professional massage therapists in movement dynamics, stress-free exercising, and Aston bodywork techniques.

▌ What's Offered

Aston-Patterning releases the built-up tensions of everyday movement and posture through the use of soft tissue massage. They also offer a line of consumer products to relieve fatigue, tension, and pain from sitting in cars or overly concave seats.

A telephone call or letter will get you their catalogue and a referral list of certified and trained Aston-Patterning practitioners.

Cranial Academy
142 West Eighth Street
Meridian, ID 83642
208-888-1201

▌ Background

The cranium, or skull, consists of eight bones joined together along hairline joints called sutures. The sutures have dovetailed, tooth-like boney material for a joint with each other. Constant movement and pressure exerted on the sutures cause them to move slightly. This movement is said to misalign and pinch the membrane covering the brain with devastating results to health.

The Cranial Academy is an educational institute for advanced training in osteopathic treatment for medical and osteopathic physicians and for dentists. This training allows them to provide extensive treatments on the cranium for such ailments as TMJ.

▌ What's Offered

Send them a self-addressed, stamped envelope, and the Cranial Academy will provide you with a referral to a member who has had extensive training in more than the usual osteopathic education in craniosacral treatment.

Federation of Straight Chiropractic Organizations
642 Broad Street
Clifton, NJ 07013
800-521-9856
201-777-1197

▌ Background

It is not uncommon that in any branch of medicine, whether orthodox or complementary, you will find splinter groups who practice a variation of what is commonly accepted.

A primary example is chiropractic. Many chiropractors use some form of kinesiology for diagnosis. Others use various therapeutic massage techniques. Still others prescribe the benefits of supplemental nutrients.

The Federation of Straight Chiropractic Organizations (FSCO) represents traditional chiropractors around the country: those who practice nontherapeutic and nondiagnostic chiropractic through vertical subluxation correction of the spine.

▌ What's Offered

If you believe that this form of chiropractic will benefit you, write or telephone the FSCO for a referral to a straight chiropractor in your area.

Feldenkrais Guild
P.O. Box 13285
Overland Park, KS 66212-3285
913-492-1444
913-492-0955 (fax)

▌ Background

The Feldenkrais Guild is an organization of physical therapists and teachers. It includes only those who have been trained by Dr. Moshe Feldenkrais or his representatives.

▌ What's Offered

Feldenkrais practitioners use a manipulative technique called functional integration. Either individually or in small groups, they teach a person's body's muscles, skeletal system, and spine to "relearn" movement with the aims of:

- ▪ Achieving balance of the nervous system
- ▪ Alleviating tremors, paralysis, ataxia, and impeded speech
- ▪ Correcting poor muscular control.

Underlying the manipulation technique is the belief that a human being's nervous system is often underdeveloped through improperly learned body movement and posture and must be retrained to achieve a "better maturation of the nervous system."

Using a series of light movements repeated 15 or 20 times, the body is taught to be more sensitive to minute changes in movement and pressure. This in turn helps to learn correct movement and posture.

A worldwide directory of qualified and accredited practitioners who are members of the Guild is published every year and will help you to locate one in your area.

A lot more Feldenkrais method information—books, audio tapes, videos, and workshop proceedings—may be obtained from the:

Feldenkrais Resources
P.O. Box 2067
Berkeley, CA 94702
800-765-1967
415-525-1907

Hellerwork, Inc.
406 Berry Street
Mount Shasta, CA 96067
800-392-3900
916-926-2500
916-926-6839 (fax)

▌ Background

Unlike other manipulative techniques, such as chiropractic or the Alexander technique, which are used in treating specific ailments, Hellerwork makes no claim to be a remedy for any specific problem. Rather, Hellerwork's deep tissue bodywork and movement education during the 11 90-minute sessions of realigning the body and releasing chronic tension and stress, are said:

- ▌ To increase energy and fitness
- ▌ To improve posture and athletic performance
- ▌ To reduce pain caused by body imbalance
- ▌ To make you look younger
- ▌ To enhance awareness of your body.

Hellerwork, Inc. was founded by Joseph Heller to train bodyworkers and therapists in his technique and is today its international headquarters and education center.

▌ What's Offered

Aside from utilizing Heller's treatment, practitioners also distribute a 32-page handbook to their clients which explains:

- ▌ The purpose of Hellerwork
- ▌ What each session will accomplish
- ▌ Exercises to do between the sessions.

When you write or telephone you will receive a geographical directory to enable you to find a practitioner in your area, as well as a short excerpt from the client's handbook which explains the principles behind Hellerwork.

Institute for Physical Fitness
P.O. Box 58
Stockbridge, MA 01262
800-221-4624
413-296-3066
413-296-3787

▌ Background

None of us can turn back the clock. None of us can go back to a time just before our pain started and do something that could have prevented it. But all of us can do something. Getting older need not mean pain and infirmity. Pain need not be a lifelong burden.

One of the newest of the manipulative therapies to relieve pain is myotherapy. The main principle behind myotherapy is that every muscle has its own trigger point that is the key to the pain in that muscle.

When a muscle's or group of muscles' trigger points start to "fire," the muscles go into spasm. Spasm causes pain, which causes more spasm, which causes more pain. To stop this spasm pain cycle, pressure is applied to the trigger points. When the pressure is released, the pain is subsided enough to allow movement or is completely gone.

Although scientists do not as yet understand the mechanism, they believe that pressure shuts down the muscle's supply of oxygen at the trigger point. Without oxygen the pain stops and the muscle relaxes.

The Institute for Physical Fitness (IPF) is associated with the School for Physical Fitness and Myotherapy that both trains and certifies myotherapists.

▌What's Offered

The Institute, founded by noted exercise and pain relief authority Bonnie Prudden, sells books, audio tapes, videos, and equipment that will show you how to find your own trigger points and apply the necessary pressure to relieve muscle pain.

From their list of certified myotherapists, the IPF will be happy to provide you with the names of fully trained and qualified myotherapists in your area.

International Chiropractic Association
1110 North Glebe Road
Suite 1000
Arlington, VA 22201
703-528-5000

▌Background

If you have ever visited a chiropractor you ubdoubtedly found many pamphlets on chiropractic—perhaps a large bound book showing research results of chiropractic case studies, perhaps a patient's newsletter.

The International Chiropractic Association (ICA) is a professional organization of chiropractors specializing in patient educational material.

▌ What's Offered

What the ICA offers to chiropractors can be purchased by anyone interested. However, the information on posture and injury prevention should be available at most chiropractors' offices.

If you regularly visit a chiropractor you will be fortunate if he or she also gets the ICA's quarterly patient newsletter, *To Your Health*. The short and lively articles on chiropractic care, sports injuries, nutrition, fitness, and prevention will take you just a few minutes to read but will be worth your time.

The ICA will also be happy to answer questions about chiropractic health care and provide you with information about consumer products that could affect your physical health and spine.

McKenzie Institute
307 East Charles Street
Muncie, IN 47305
800-635-8380
317-289-3979
317-288-6656 (fax)

▌ Background

Many manipulative techniques to relieve spinal or spine-related pain exist. Chiropractic, osteopathy, and orthopaedic medicine are the best-known in America.

A new method of diagnosing and treating nonspecific spinal pain, developed in New Zealand by physiotherapist Robin McKenzie, is now available in the United States. The McKenzie method's treatment goals are to eliminate pain, restore full function, and prevent recurrence and progression of the problem.

The treatment method consists of a series of exercises that are specific to the sufferer's disorder and education in posture, movement, and prevention. The exercises that are effective become the focus of treatment, with new exercises added to assure that recovery is complete. In essence, the McKenzie therapist teaches the patient how to treat his or her own neck and back problems and how to minimize the risk of and deal with recurrence.

The McKenzie Institute, founded to teach the methods of Robin McKenzie:

- Disseminates information to the public and health care profession on the methods
- Assures that the method is available to patients by qualified practitioners
- Supports and conducts research on the method and its practice.

What's Offered

The Institute provides clinical training to professionals, certifies the professional competence of practitioners, and distributes the self-help books and specially designed back pillows of Robin McKenzie.

Further information and a referral to a professional in your area may be obtained by writing or telephoning.

North American Academy of Musculoskeletal Medicine
7611 Elmwood Avenue
Suite 202
Middleton, WI 53562
608-831-9240
608-831-5122 (fax)

Background

All manipulative techniques use the hands to apply mechanical force to various parts of the body. In general, all these techniques are used to diagnose and treat functional disorders of the mechanical and soft tissue system or to restore and enhance neuromusculoskeletal functions.

The North American Academy of Musculoskeletal Medicine (NAAM) is a professional organization of all types of licensed physicians practicing musculoskeletal diagnosis and treatment. It provides continuing education and certification in various modalities of manipulative medicine and a network for peer consultation.

▌ What's Offered

NAAM's eight-page, quarterly newsletter, *The Touchstone*, presents short case histories, information on certification, extracts from other publications, book reviews, and news of upcoming events.

Of more importance to the consumer, NAAM also provides a referral service of its members.

North American Society of Teachers of the Alexander Technique
P.O. Box 3992
Champaign, IL 61826-3992
217-359-3529

▌ Background

Like many manipulative techniques, practitioners of the Alexander technique believe that muscular habits account for much of the physical tension many of us feel. Rarely noticed because we are so accustomed to it, this tension interferes with healthy mental and physical functioning.

The Alexander technique teaches you to use the right amount of energy for each particular activity through a series of simple movements involving the simplest of tasks: sitting, walking, or even talking. Old habits are changed through practice, and internal feedback systems make them new habits over time.

The North American Society of Teachers of the Alexander Technique (NASTAT) provides educational material on the Alexander technique and establishes and maintains standards for certification for both practitioners and trainers.

▌ What's Offered

Several pamphlets discussing the basis of the Alexander technique methodology and benefits to be derived from the treatment are avaliable.

Upon request, NASTAT will also send you a national directory of certified Alexander technique teachers from which you will be able to find one in your area.

Rolf Institute
P.O. Box 1868
Boulder, CO 80306
303-449-5903

▌ Background

We have all seen people who don't stand up straight, but seem to favor one side or hunch forward. Others sit in a chair in an awkward position, bending to the right or left.

Rolfing is a connective tissue manipulation technique designed to bring the body's major segments—head, shoulders, thorax, pelvis, and legs—toward vertical alignment.

The Rolf Institute is an organization of physical therapists and teachers. It includes those who have been trained by Dr. Ida P. Rolf or her representatives.

▌ What's Offered

Rolf professionals use a manipulative technique called structural integration to overcome the effects of the pull of gravity on the major segments of the body. It takes place in a series of 10 sessions and proceeds from the skin's surface toward deeper and deeper local areas of muscular contraction and displacement. Force is applied to stretch and move tissues in order to overcome their accumulated tension. The force often results in some soreness, and pain frequently occurs when the tensions are released. The aim of Rolfing is:

- To improve balance
- To alleviate tension and the emotional stress in the body's muscles and deep tissues
- To release the physical and psychological memory of trauma
- To increase muscle efficiency.

Several books, article reprints, and training schedules are available from the Rolf Institute along with a free international directory of qualified and accredited Rolfers to help you to locate a Rolfer in your area.

Trager Institute
10 Old Mill Road
Mill Valley, CA 94941-1891
415-388-2688

Contact: Don Scwartz, Ph.D.

▌ Background

Relaxation. Everyone clamors to relieve tensions and reduce stress, or, in other words, to relax.

The Trager method—developed by Dr. Milton Trager—is a system of very gentle, rhythmic, nonintrusive movements performed on someone by a certified specialist. The result of a session facilitates deep relaxation and increases physical mobility and mental clarity. Said to release deep-seated physical or mental restrictions, Trager is said to be both a physical as well as a psychological therapy.

The Trager Institute offers certification programs in the Trager method.

▍ What's Offered

A Trager session, called a psychological integration session, involves a very special kind of physical contact. There are no oils or lotions, no violent, jerky movements, no effort exerted. All sessions include lessons in mentastics, a system of movement sequences, developed to enhance the benefits of the Trager sessions, that you can do on your own.

The Institute will be happy to provide you with referrals to certified Trager practitioners in your area.

Further Resources
    see all resources under ORIENTAL HEALING AND EXERCISE
    American College of Sports Medicine
    New York Open Center, Inc.

PARENTING

Childhood
RR1
P.O. Box 2675
Westford, VT 05494
802-879-4869

Contact: Nancy Aldrich

▌ Background

Many sources of information on child rearing exist. Indeed, there seems to be a new one sprouting up daily. More and more of them are taking a fresh look at children; many present a holistic, well-rounded view of parenting.

Childhood stands out from the crowd. It focuses exclusively on the Waldorf philosphy of child development. Waldorf's viewpoint seeks to promote home schooling and to develop an intuitive approach to parenting.

▌ What's Offered

Childhood is a 42-page, almost handcrafted, quarterly ($24). Articles are offset by drawings and sketches. Reader surveys help the magazine to have a warm and friendly personality. Many articles are on handcrafting, and each issue contains reviews of children's books, especially those that seek to teach. Some topics from several recent issues are:

- Education—gifted children
- Music—children's experience

- Music and mathematics books for children
- Five-year-olds
- Cognitive development—early childhood education
- Home schooling
- Intuition in children
- Childhood and spiritual origins
- Cycles of learning
- Storytelling.

Several information packets on the Waldorf philosophy are also available.

La Leche League International
9616 Minneapolis Avenue
P.O. Box 1209
Franklin Park, IL 60131-8209
800-LA-LECHE
708-455-7730

▌ Background

Breast milk is unquestionably the best source of nutrition for a newborn baby.

The La Leche League International believes that breastfeeding offers physical and emotional benefits for both mother and baby. They conduct physicians' seminars and workshops and provide a large catalogue of books, reprints, and pamphlets on breastfeeding and other health matters.

▌ What's Offered

A $25 yearly membership in La Leche includes a subscription to the 32-page, bimonthly *New Beginnings* magazine, containing articles on breastfeeding and mother-to-mother information.

Their extensive catalogue includes many hard-to-find items and will provide you and your health care practitioner with all the information on this subject available.

Mothering
P.O. Box 1690
Santa Fe, NM 87504
505-984-8116

▌ Background

The baby boomers are having babies themselves. Births are up, and parenting has replaced disco dancing as the thing to do.

Mothering as a part of parenting, whether an alternative or mainstream philosophy is followed, means more than giving birth to and feeding a newborn.

Mothering, a quarterly ($18), presents ideas, news, and viewpoints on parenting (both mothers and fathers) from a concern about the rise of cesareans to questioning routine vaccinations for children.

▌ What's Offered

Professionally put together and written by experts with a broad range of viewpoints, *Mothering* always includes many regular features and articles on a wide variety of topics. There is often a readers' survey and always letters to the editor. The articles are written by respected authorities in their field and are quite comprehensive; they are often a tutorial on the subject. Many of the authors may be contacted for further information. A partial list of some topics covered in the last few issues includes:

- ▪ Holding your baby

- Homeopathy for children
- Ear infections in babies
- Doctor–patient communication
- Phototherapy
- Breastfeeding benefits
- Home schooling
- Miscarriages
- Violence and spanking
- Video display terminals and pregnancy
- Immunization
- Breastfeeding and sexuality
- Dangers of vaccinations.

Back issues, a few books on parenting, and several audio tapes are available as well.

Pediatrics for Parents
P.O. Box 1069
Bangor, ME 04402-1069
207-942-6212
207-947-3134 (fax)

▌ Background

Everyone agrees that from the moment they're born, most American kids really have it good. Most newborns have their very own doctors: pediatricians. Most of them get to see their pediatrician routinely, even for trivial health matters.

Pediatrics for Parents is a 10-page, monthly ($18) newsletter that helps parents get through the maze of health information on children. It believes that well-informed parents have healthier and happier children.

▌ What's Offered

Although not written entirely from an alternative health perspective, this newsletter does seek to provide parents with timely, practical information about their children's health. Articles come from a variety of sources. Some are excerpted from scientific and medical journals, others are written by experts in the field of child development or health. All are fact-filled and cover their topic completely. Some recent topics covered are:

- Breathing problems—family histories
- Fevers—treatments
- Ear infections—vaccines
- Bed-wetting—help
- Tantrums
- Twins
- Screening for lead poisoning.

Priority Parenting
Priority Parenting Publications
P.O. Box 1793
Warsaw, IN 46580-1793
219-453-3864

Contact: Tamra B. Orr, Editor

▌ Background

Published monthly ($14), the 12-page *Priority Parenting* magazine encourages natural childcare. Rather than short summaries of a number of topics, each issue is devoted to a single topic and is thoroughly explored.

▌ What's Offered

Besides focusing on its one topic, each issue features book, tape, and video reviews; announcements of upcoming parenting conferences, workshops, and seminars; and a readers' column for parents and children to network among themselves. The main topic is discussed from many perspectives. Some articles are personal, others scientific and replete with references. All are literate and present much food for thought on that topic. Issues discussed have included:

- ▌ Spirituality in the home
- ▌ Miscarriage
- ▌ Adoption
- ▌ Drugs and children
- ▌ Midwifery
- ▌ Environmental concerns for parents.

Further Resources
Positive Pregnancy & Parenting Fitness

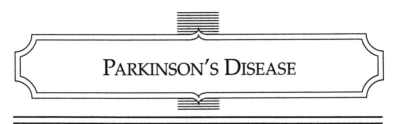

PARKINSON'S DISEASE

Parkinson's Education Program
3900 Birch Street
Suite 105
Newport Beach, CA 92660
800-344-7872
714-250-2975
714-250-8530 (fax)

▌ Background

Parkinson's disease affects close to 750,000 Americans. It is a central nervous system disorder of unknown cause that leads to the characteristic symptoms of trembling of the limbs, increased resistance to passive movement, and excessive slowness of bodily movement.

The Parkinson's Education Program (PEP) cannot by the wildest stretch of the imagination be categorized as an alternative health care resource. Yet, its two mottos—"Information Brings Awareness" and "Help Yourself, Help Your Loved Ones"—and its primary aim—to assist Parkinson's sufferers and their families—make it mandatory that it be included in this directory.

PEP's stated aims are:

- To promote support groups and assist them with information
- To act as an advocate to protect the rights of patients
- To educate the public to understand Parkinsonism
- To encourage and support the education of health care professionals
- To promote research for causes and therapies
- To provide counseling for patients.

▌ What's Offered

PEP publishes a four-page, monthly ($15) newsletter, *PEP Exchange*. Its articles include information about medication used to treat parkinsonism, updates on current research, book reviews, hints and tips for patients and their families, and coping and psychological support.

An extensive catalogue offers books and pamphlets on Parkinson's disease, exercise for patients, nutritional information, support groups, research and treatment data, audio tapes, and videos.

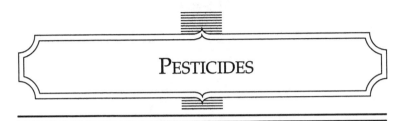

PESTICIDES

Americans for Safe Food
Center for Science in the Public Interest
1501 16th Street, NW
Washington, DC 20036
202-332-9110

Contact: Roger Blobaum, Project Director

▌ Background

You are what you eat is a pithy truism. But what if what you eat contains residues of pesticides, additives, dangerous preservatives, and drugs given to animals? You still will be what you eat.

Americans for Safe Food (ASF) focuses its efforts on the many potentially harmful additives, pesticides, and drugs used to produce our food.

▌ What's Offered

ASF will send you a free list of mail-order firms selling organic produce and other food products. You may also help procure locally grown organic produce in supermarkets with their effort and help shape public policy toward food and agriculture.

National Coalition Against the Misuse of Pesticides
701 E Street, SE
Suite 200
Washington, DC 20003
202-543-5450

Contact: Kathryn Martin

▋ Background

Almost all the produce in the United States is grown with the use of pesticides. Many people believe that pesticides are safe because they are registered by the U.S. Environmental Protection Agency (EPA) and used according to their labels.

However, a 1982 congressional report concluded that between 79% and 84% of pesticides in use have not been adequately tested for carcinogens; 80% to 93% have not been tested for their ability to cause genetic damage; and 60% to 70% have not been tested for their ability to cause birth defects. Furthermore, a 1984 National Academy of Science report stated that only 10% of all registered pesticide formulations have been analyzed for health hazards.

The National Coalition Against the Misuse of Pesticides, a grass-roots network whose primary goal is to make people more aware of pesticide dangers, is also engaged in educating the general public about the use of pesticides in schools and lawns and about other pest-control matters.

▋ What's Offered

The Coalition also offers information on safe alternatives to pest control and publishes its newsletter, *Pesticides and You*, five times a year ($20). Several brochures, booklets, monographs, and technical reports are also available. Some of the topics covered are:

    ▪ Lawns—least toxic methods of pest control

- Pesticides in fruits and vegetables
- Pesticide safety
- EPA food residue estimates—reliability
- Pesticide resistance
- Drinking water—safety
- Commercial agriculture—soil erosion and pesticides.

National Pesticide Telecommunications Network
Texas Tech University Health Sciences Center
School of Medicine
Department of Preventive Medicine and Community Health
Lubbock, TX 79430
800-858-PEST
806-743-3094 (fax)

Background

Pesticides abound. Hundreds of new ones are introduced every year. It is next to impossible to find out what the active ingredients are and whether you exhibit known symptoms of being poisoned.

The National Pesticide Telecommunications Network (NPTN) was set up to disseminate accurate and prompt information about pesticides to anyone in the United States, 24 hours a day, 365 days a year.

What's Offered

Your telephone call will be taken by a pesticide specialist: graduate students in the fields of biology, anatomy, biochemistry, and entomology. NPTN maintains its own library on toxicity, human and environmental effects, and proper use of each pesticide, cross-referenced by trade name, chemical name, generic name, and manufacturer's name. Additionally, NPTN is connected via computer to the National Library of Medicine's MEDLINE and TOX-LINE databases.

The kinds of information you can get include:

- Pesticide product information
- Symptom and toxicity information
- Safety information
- Health and environmental effects
- Poisoning recognition and management
- Referrals for emergency treatments.

Natural Resources Defense Council
40 West 20th Street
New York, NY 10114-0466
212-727-2700

▋ Background

Whether one believes that pesticides help protect the public from tainted food and assure its widespread availablity or that they are deadly toxins that harm us all, it is only through rigorous scientific evaluation that one can reach an objective conclusion.

The Natural Resources Defense Council (NRDC) is a non-profit organization striving to protect natural resources and to improve the quality of food through the reduction or elimination of toxic substances. The NRDC prepares and distributes scientifically based information.

▋ What's Offered

Aside from much work on environmental issues and the publication of *The American Journal*, the NRDC has prepared a number of reports on food hazards and pesticides including:

- Pesticides in children's food
- Protection against pesticides
- Meat and poultry—hidden hazards
- Fruits and vegetables.

PREVENTION

Alternatives For The Health Conscious Individual
Mountain Home Publishing
P.O. Box 829
Ingram, TX 78025
512-367-4492

Contact: Dr. David G. Williams, Editor

▮ Background

Mountain Home Publishing publishes the monthly ($39) *Alternatives For The Health Conscious Individual* as well as a number of books by Dr. David G. Williams.

▮ What's Offered

The eight-page newsletter is devoted to providing health information on alternative treatments for diseases and their prevention through a more natural lifestyle in the areas of diet and exercise. All articles include technical information, practical advice, sources where further information or products may be obtained, and scientific references. Letters to the editor and readers' tips offer follow-up and practical suggestions of recently published stories. Recent issues have included articles on:

- Flavinoids
- Enzyme therapy
- Parkinson's disease
- Alzheimer's disease and drugs
- Olive oil and cholesterol

- Selenium deficiency
- Magnesium sulfate infusions and heart attacks
- Allergies and hyperactivity
- Cataract treatment with bilberry extract
- Understanding the immune system.

Books and reports on a variety of health-related subjects have included:

- Life extension
- Herpes and BHT
- Infant mortality
- Metabolic balancing
- Back issues of the newsletter.

American College of Preventive Medicine
1015 15th Street, NW
Suite 403
Washington, DC 20005
202-789-0003

▌ Background

It is axiomatic that an important part of alternative health care is prevention of illness. But part of mainstream medicine is also interested in this alternative health practice.

The stated mission of the American College of Preventive Medicine (ACPM) is to preserve and promote good health; to prevent disease, injury, and disability; and to facilitate early diagnosis and treatment of illness.

▌ What's Offered

While membership is open only to professionals, ACPM's publications are available to everyone. It publishes the bimonthly magazine, *ACPM News*, containing newsy articles about the ACPM and what it is doing.

The scholarly, academic, and highly technical bimonthly, *The American Journal of Preventive Medicine*, is also published under its auspices. In it you will find original articles, book reviews, critical commentaries, editorials, and technical correspondence. A recent sponsored professional conference included the following topics:

- Politics of prevention
- Community empowerment
- Chronic disease prevention
- Sports and exercise.

A membership directory may be purchased. In it you should be able to find a medical physician in your area whose practice focuses on prevention rather than after-the-fact treatment.

American Health Federation
One Dana Road
Valhalla, NY 10595
914-592-2600

Contact: Deborah Holder

▌ Background

The major chronic diseases—cancer, heart disease, and stroke—account for one American death a minute. Over two-thirds of them could be prevented by switching from after-the-fact medical care to prevention.

The American Health Federation does basic laboratory research to find the causes and mechanisms of these diseases. As part of its educational mission and to help fund research, it is engaged in public education through the publication of *Health Letter*, a bimonthly ($15), eight-page newsletter.

▌What's Offered

Health Letter divides its short, easy-to-read articles into the topics of health research, prevention, nutrition, public health, health behavior, and news briefs. Some recent topics have included:

- Reading food labels
- Determining your cancer risks
- Nutrition and breakfast
- Salad bars—how healthy are they?
- Aging research.

A number of inexpensive brochures and pamphlets on cholesterol, children's menus, and snack foods written for the general public are also available.

Bestways
Bestways Magazine, Inc.
P.O. Box 570
Oak Park, IL 60303
312-848-8100
312-848-9175 (fax)

▌Background

Bestways, a colorful, monthly ($18) magazine, stresses a holistic down-to-earth, preventive approach for the health-minded individual.

▮ What's Offered

Articles cover health, fitness, nutrition, Eastern and Western medicine, herbalism, nutrient supplementation, and healthy eating. All are written by professionals and educators and are presented as practical advice rather than as theoretical information. There are several worthwhile monthly features on health: answers to readers' health questions, recipes for health, natural beauty, and health and medical news. Recent articles have covered:

- Yoga and massage—stress reduction and pain relief
- Fluoridation—effects on behavior
- Advances in supplements—vitamins and minerals
- Protecting yourself from the harmful effects of air pollution and environmental radiation
- Wellness and homeopathy
- Exercising in the office
- Aloe vera and the immune system
- Barley to combat cholesterol
- Cooking with eggplant.

Better Nutrition for Today's Living
Communication Channels, Inc.
6255 Barfield Road
Atlanta, GA 30328
404-256-9800

▮ Background

Better Nutrition for Today's Living is a monthly ($12), full-color magazine usually found at the checkout counters in health food stores; it is often given to customers without charge.

▋ What's Offered

Better Nutrition's articles are free from jargon, not overly burdened with theory, and usually well researched. More often than not they're illustrated, have quotes from well-known experts and scientific journals, mention case histories, give practical advice for implementation, and have numerous references and citations from the world literature. Regular monthly columns on recipes, nutritional therapies for illnesses and ongoing research, nutrition hotline, book reviews, and new product news add to the magazine's interest. In all, this magazine is a fast read. Recent articles have included information on:

- Anemia
- Nutrient therapy for skin ailments
- PMS herbal products
- Boron—an essential trace element
- Colds and homeopathy
- Spirulina and nutrition
- Colds and flu
- Folic acid and spina bifida
- Natural digestive aids
- Garlic and circulation
- Insomnia treatments using herbs
- Pau d'arco for the immune system
- Sports nutrition and training.

Cooking for Survival Consciousness
P.O. Box 26762
Elkins Park, PA 19117
215-635-1022

Contact: Beatrice Wittels

▌ Background

As it relates to your health, you are what you eat, breathe, and think. Cooking for Survival Consciousness (CSC) concerns itself with what you eat. Its primary focus is disseminating information on:

- ▌ Preventive health care through nutrition and diet
- ▌ Diet-linked disease and prevention
- ▌ Alternative approaches to nutrition.

▌ What's Offered

Annual membership ($25) includes a subscription to *CSC Report*, a quarterly, tabloid-sized, 20-page newspaper. The short and practical articles will give you an overview of their topics along with citations for follow-up study and resources to contact. Recent article topics have included:

- ▌ Electromagnetic radiation
- ▌ Water—contamination
- ▌ Chinese nutrition
- ▌ Computer safety
- ▌ Gardening
- ▌ Food irradiation
- ▌ Enzymes.

CSC sells a variety of enzymatic nutrients to support its research and conducts several seminars on alternative viewpoints in human nutrition.

Council for Responsible Nutrition
1300 19th Street, NW
Suite 310
Washington, DC 20036-1609
202-872-1488
202-872-9594 (fax)

▌Background

It's clear that most Americans do not even get the minimum daily allowances set forth by the government. Furthermore, many nutrients are not even mentioned in the guidelines, and the benefits of larger doses are considered medical advice and thus forbidden to appear on labels.

The Council for Responsible Nutrition (CRN) cannot, by the wildest stretch of the imagination, be said to be alternative. Rather, it is a trade association representing manufacturers and distributors of nutrient supplements. Nevertheless, the information available from it is accurate and useful.

▌What's Offered

The CRN will send you a rather extensive package. Much of the information concerns itself with the trade practices of nutrient manufacturers and distributors and the legislature they would like to see enacted with respect to labeling and health claims on nutrients.

However, included along with that will also be much information on the benefits of nutritional supplements for the elderly, children, pregnant women, smokers, dieters, and most other people, along with the positive benefits many nutritional supplements can have in protecting against major diseases. The information is abstracted from scientific journals, monographs, bibliographies, texts, and magazines.

Delicious
New Hope Communications
1301 Spruce Street
Boulder, CO 8302
303-939-8440
303-939-9559 (fax)

▌ Background

Delicious, published monthly ($17), is, in the words of its publishers, "designed to educate consumers about healthy living." A 50-page, full-color magazine, you will often find it at the checkout counters in health food stores where it is often given away without charge.

▌ What's Offered

Like other magazines of this type, *Delicious* offers its readers health information in easy-to-swallow doses. Unlike the other magazines, these articles are shorter, have more razzle-dazzle graphics, and are filled with practical tidbits in sidebars. All the information has a distinct environmental twist. Monthly departments are on health and nutrition news, natural healing, and new products. A nice touch to the recipes is the information on fat and cholesterol percentages. Some recent topics have included:

- ▌ Vitamin E for the heart
- ▌ Herbs for allergies
- ▌ Natural hair care
- ▌ Nutrition and hormones
- ▌ Flu and homeopathic remedies
- ▌ Ginkgo biloba for immunity
- ▌ Drinking-water standards
- ▌ Protecting your eyes with natural remedies
- ▌ Chinese herbal medicine
- ▌ Ayurvedic medicine

- Women's herbs
- Japanese cuisine
- Breakfast recipes for energy.

Edell Health Letter
Hippocrates, Inc.
475 Gate Five Road
Suite 225
Sausalito, CA 94965
415-332-5866

Background

Even if you wished to get the latest health information, going through medical journals and health publications would be a full-time job. That's the main reason for the popularity of many health publications that present medical and health news summaries.

That's exactly what *Edell Health Letter* does. However, by no means is this an alternative health care publication. Rather, as the evidence in peer-reviewed journals reports the benefits of nutrition and a lifestyle stressing prevention, more and more of this magazine's stories do the same.

What's Offered

Subscriptions are $24 for this monthly newsletter. It contains the latest medical discoveries, new theories of disease causes and prevention, and debates over medical findings. The information is taken from over 150 medical journals and health news publications. The very short articles—summaries, really—also include references. They are soberly written without being overly technical. Examples of topics covered in the past are:

- Aspirin and the heart—aspirin's blood-thinning abilities bad for people at risk for macular degeneration
- The mystery in cholesterol numbers
- The problems with blood pressure measurements—physician's testing equipment not maintained for accuracy
- High animal-protein diets and bone weakness—animal protein leaches calcium from bones
- Zinc supplements and macular degeneration—a simple cure and means of prevention
- Low-fat diets and cancer protection—less fat lowers estrogen and testosterone.

Environmental Nutrition
2112 Broadway
Suite 200
New York, NY 10023
212-362-0424

▌ Background

Environmental Nutrition, calling itself "The Professional Newsletter of Diet, Nutrition and Health," is a monthly ($28) newsletter that believes that nutrition consists in not only what we eat, but in how, when, and where we eat. Its stated mission is:

- To bring you nutritional research information affecting overall health
- To inform you of pharmaceutical, vitamin, amd mineral updates
- To tell you what to avoid in foods
- To critique the most popular diets and food fads.

▮ What's Offered

Under the four broad topics of vitamin and mineral research, popular misconceptions, chemicals in food, and dietary link to illness, all the lively and well-presented articles will keep you informed in just a few easily digested pages. Examples of information recently seen include:

- Foods to control fat and cholesterol
- Relationship of food to chronic illness
- Food allergy myths
- New foods and products
- Fiber guidelines
- Food nutritional ratings
- Grapefruit pectin (fibrous membranes found in the pulp)—reduces the formation of artery-clogging plaque.

Back issues and a variety of booklets on nutrition, diet, and nutritional therapies for major and chronic diseases can also be ordered.

Executive Health Report
80 Enterprise Way
P.O. Box 8880
Chapel Hill, NC 27515-8880
919-929-7519
919-929-2458 (fax)

▮ Background

We all have our own picture of an executive. Whatever that picture is, it is likely to be that of a man—a man out of shape. No longer as universal as it once was, the picture still remains an all too-true view of many American businessmen.

Executive Health Report, an eight-page, monthly $34 newsletter, reports on new health and medical findings for the busy executive.

▌ What's Offered

Stressing prevention, this newsletter's short articles offer practical advice. All the articles are written by physicians or other health care practitioners and present information from a variety of scientific sources. Issues include regular columns, readers' questions and answers, wellness tips from medical publications, exercising, and nutrition. Topics discussed from several issues are:

- Running—pros and cons
- Chronic pain and illness
- Cancer and emotions
- Baldness
- Stress and the rat race
- Vitamin E—disease prevention and natural sources
- Emotions and the body.

Foundation for Innovation in Medicine
411 North Avenue East
Cranford, NJ 07016
908-272-2967
908-272-4583 (fax)

Contact: Patricia A. Park, Director of Administration

▌ Background

No one can deny any longer that nutrients can help prevent illnesses and promote their cures. That's one of the reasons why some foods are better for you than others. For example, grapefruit pectin, carotenoids, flavinoids, terpenes, and liminoids help lower cholesterol. This, in turn, helps fight cancer and heart disease. Cruciferous vegetables such as broccoli are recommended by even conservative physicians and medical groups for their beta carotene, which has been shown to prevent cancer.

But using nutrients themselves to prevent or treat illness still remains an underground activity. Manufacturers and distributors are forbidden by law to claim any health or medical benefits. Many physicians are not even aware of the studies that support such claims.

The Foundation for Innovation in Medicine encourages research in the use of nutriceuticals: nutritional substances with pharmaceutical properties. It also seeks to change the regulations regarding the labeling of these products, enabling them to be recognized as having valid therapeutic benefits.

▌What's Offered

While no immediate and direct benefits are available from the Foundation's work to change the FDA's regulations, writing will bring you several articles on its work and information on which nutrients show medical promise in disease prevention and cure.

Healing Currents
Tapestry Press
P.O. Box 653
Springville, UT 84663
800-333-4290

▌Background

Healing Currents, a bimonthly ($10), is a series of 16- to 24-page booklets on a single health-related topic written from an alternative health perspective.

▌ What's Offered

Not only a lively introduction to some of the thinking on complementary medicine and alternative views on health, each issue also presents the point of view of its author, Dean Black, Ph.D.

A condensation of much of the available research on its topic, each booklet is also full of practical, easy-to-apply information. For example, the booklet on the Chinese theory of regenerative healing, discusses not only the principles of natural healing but gives specific formulations of herbs and how they can help.

A few of the past booklet topics include:

- Chinese healing principles
- Food additive problems
- Chronic fatigue syndrome
- Mercury dental fillings
- Immunization
- Vitamin C
- PMS and the loss of natural body rhythms
- Educated persons and natural healing
- Diet and behavior
- Candida.

Several of Black's books, audio tapes, and videos are also available.

Health and Healing
Phillips Publishing, Inc.
7811 Montrose Road
P.O. Box 59745
Potomac, MD 20854
800-777-5005
301-340-2647 (fax)

▌ Background

Your physician's job is not to keep you healthy; it's to make you healthy when you get sick. Like most people, doctors have fears, and two of them could kill you. Terrified of malpractice suits, doctors will often perform many unnecessary tests and prescribe unnecessary treatments and drugs, just to cover themselves. And, like most other people, they don't want to be called nonconformist by seeking the approval of their peers—in this case, other doctors.

The monthly ($39) *Health and Healing* offers information on preventing illness through lifestyle changes and self-help alternative therapies for common ailments.

▌ What's Offered

A new and exclusively alternative health care information source, *Health and Healing* is edited by Dr. Julian Whitaker, a leading advocate of safer and alternative approaches to health care. A monthly feature is the column by Jane Heimlich, noted author of several books on alternative health care.

Like other publications of this company, the newsletter articles are lively and eclectic, taking you less than an hour to finish. There are few technical terms, less jargon, and no lengthy, theoretical explanations. Instead, practical advice on common, everyday complaints, problems, and illnesses is offered. Topics covered are:

- Vitamins and supplements to help your body fight disease
- Creating the best exercise program for yourself
- Reversing the effects of disease without drugs or surgery
- Being a wise medical consumer
- Private health insurance risks
- Vegetables that heal
- Dangers of so-called light junk foods
- Disease-proofing your body
- Foods that make your body burn fat
- Tapping into your own body's natural healing powers.

Health Consciousness
P.O. Box 550
Oviedo, FL 32765
407-365-6681
407-365-1834 (fax)

Background

Health Consciousness is a 72-page, bimonthly ($30), colorful maga-
zine, stressing holistic health from the viewpoint of its publisher,
Dr. Roy Kupsinel.

What's Offered

Articles cover health, the environment, guest editorials by alternative healers, news of alternative treatments from other countries,
book reviews, and news of upcoming alternative health events.
The information is always well-researched and intelligently presented, although lacking in references and citations for further
study. Recent article topics have included:

- The safety of distilled water
- Love and psychological balance
- European perspectives on food hygiene
- Viral vaccines—safety and vulnerability
- The efficacy of feng-shui
- Dental pain control
- Mercury filling toxicity.

Health News & Review
Keats Publishing, Inc.
27 Pine Street
P.O. Box 876
New Canaan, CT 06840-0876
203-966-8721

Background

Health News & Review is part of the growing number of sources for health and disease prevention available to the general public. Unlike its competitors, it is a tabloid-sized newspaper rather than a slick and glossy full-color magazine.

What's Offered

A subscription to the bimonthly ($12) *Health News & Review* brings you a wide variety of short articles on current health topics of interest. Regular features include book reviews and excerpts from other health and medical publications. Some recent topics covered have been:

- New uses for vitamin E—cataracts, cancer
- Green food—spirulina, chlorella, green barley
- Minerals and health
- Herbal remedies—women only
- Facial exercises—muscle toning
- Irritable bowel syndrome—lactose
- Microwave oven safety
- Elusive chemical sensitivities
- Memory and nutrition
- Naturopath—choosing one
- Mercury fillings.

International Academy of Nutrition and Preventive Medicine
P.O. Box 18433
Asheville, NC 28814-0433
704-258-3243

Contact: Carroll Thompson, Executive Director

▌ Background

There is an old saw about an ounce of prevention being worth a pound of cure. That's a 16-to-1 advantage in favor of prevention. An integral part of anybody's health prevention plan should be nutrition.

The International Academy of Nutrition and Preventive Medicine (IANPM) is dedicated to promoting prevention and nutrition education for professionals and laypersons.

▌ What's Offered

A $20 membership fee to IANPM will bring you the bimonthly, eight-page newsletter, *Your Health*, with short practical health care articles, book reviews, and organization news. Some recent articles have discussed:

- Quality preconceptual care
- Sources of cholesterol
- Natural headache relief with acupressure
- Natural reduction of arterial plaque.

The IANPM's premier publication is the biannual ($20) *Journal of Applied Nutrition*. In it you will find scientific reports and reviews, case studies, commentaries, editorials, book reviews, abstracts of other articles, and correspondence from professionals. But its main thrust is the original research articles that stress the practical applications of nutrition and preventive medicine. A refereed journal, it is open to ideas that often have difficulty finding a forum in mainstream, academic journals.

- Diet and lifestyle influences on cochlear disorders
- Aspartame reactions—case study of 551 persons
- Chronic dental pain and food restriction
- Food allergies and autism
- L-carnitine metabolism and human nutrition.

IANPM also maintains an information-referral service open to anyone seeking to find a preventive, nutrition-oriented health care professional in his or her local community.

Let's Live
444 North Larchmont Boulevard
Los Angeles, CA 90004
213-469-3900

▌ Background

Let's Live, a 48-page, full-color monthly ($12.95) magazine, offers practical advice for the health-minded individual.

▌ What's Offered

Articles span the spectrum of health, medicine, alternative treatments, recipes for the health-minded, news of health and medicine, and book reviews. All are served up in an informal but informative manner. Many of the articles give references for further study. Experts in the field are often quoted or called on to write on the subject themselves. Regular monthly features on natural beauty, pet care, readers' questions, environmental concerns, and medical news are lively one-page summaries of the latest information on each topic covered. Recent articles have discussed:

- Nutrients and longevity
- PMS—herbal and nutrient treatments
- Eczema—herbal products
- Choosing a doctor
- Vitamin E and brain damage
- Nutrient deficiencies in the elderly
- Chemicals commonly found in hair conditioners
- Cholesterol and chromium polynicotinate
- Arthritis in household pets.

Macrobiotics Today
George Ohsawa Macrobiotic Foundation
1151 Robinson Street
Oroville, CA 95965
916-533-7702

▌ Background

The relationship between diet and health is now an accepted fact, even among the most stalwart of the medical community. Macrobiotics consists of a specific vegetarian regimen consisting primarily of brown rice, soy foods, sea vegetables, teas, and condiments. If adopted in part or whole, it can contribute to the dietary goals of a high-carbohydrate, low-fat, low-cholesterol, low-sugar, low-salt diet.

Macrobiotics Today, a 40-page bimonthly ($15) magazine, is the major publication of the George Ohsawa Macrobiotic Foundation, a leading advocate and research institute in macrobiotics.

▌ What's Offered

Written in a straightforward, no-nonsense style, the magazine will provide you with continuing information about macrobiotics and a macrobiotic lifestyle. Some sample topics covered in recent issues are:

- ▮ Medicine and macrobiotics
- ▮ Biomechanical mechanisms of macrobiotics
- ▮ Macrobiotic recipes
- ▮ Organic growing
- ▮ National directory of macrobiotic centers and health food stores.

Natural Health
P.O. Box 1200
Brookline Village, MA 02147
617-232-1000

▌ Background

Joining what appears to be the already overcrowded field of health publications requires a high degree of confidence that what you have to say is different from the others.

Natural Health: The Guide to Well-Being, believes that its message is different.

▌ What's Offered

The bimonthly ($11.97) *Natural Health* looks, at first glance, like every other magazine believing itself to promote good health. Glossy and colorful, its articles look timely. The usual emotion-evoking words such as *natural* and *holistic* appear frequently. But that's where the similarities end. The differences are its consistency and the care taken to present its message. The thoroughly researched articles contain much that may not be found in the usual fare of magazines. The information given blends theory and practicality and leaves you feeling that it was worth reading. The recipes discuss more than ingredients, food preparation, and ultimate taste: They talk knowledgeably about nutrition and the reason behind the food combining. Topics discussed from several recent issues include:

- Choosing a holistic health care professional
- Herbal remedies—building natural defenses to illness
- Cures and remissions—case studies
- Natural sweeteners—differences and similarities to sugar
- Food combining—digestion, absorption of nutrients
- Birth control—women's viewpoint
- Eyesight—natural ways to improve vision
- Homeopathy—cold and flu remedies
- Air pollution—building the body's defenses.

Natural Lifestyle and Your Health
KPI Publishing
P.O. Box 278
Pine River, WI 54965-0278
414-987-5866

▌ Background

Natural Lifestyle and Your Health, a monthly ($15), 12-page newsletter, in its own words "offers practical answers to how your lifestyle affects your health."

▌ What's Offered

Like many others discussed in this book, this newsletter presents short articles of easy-to-follow advice. Unlike a few others, the research done is reinforced with references following many of the articles. In fact, a great deal of the "medical" material is written by complementary physicians and includes follow-up references and citations. Lifestyle articles are written by professional journalists, and recipes are usually from a selection of cookbooks specializing in healthful eating. A sample of the articles from a few recent issues are:

- ▪ Lifestyles to reverse diseases
- ▪ Chronic fatigue syndrome—diet and nutritional treatments
- ▪ Recipes—vegetarian
- ▪ Herbal preparations for treating minor maladies
- ▪ Diabetes prevention through diet and nutrients
- ▪ Headache relief
- ▪ Sprouting to increase the nutrients in plants
- ▪ Cancer and stress
- ▪ Digestion.

Natural Living Newsletter
NLN Publications, Inc.
P.O. Box 849
Madison Square Station
New York, NY 10159

▌ Background

Natural Living Newsletter, a four-page newsletter published (more or less) monthly ($28), presents the findings and research of Gary Null, Ph.D., author of many books on alternative health care, lifestyles, and prevention and the host of several radio health shows.

▌ What's Offered

Perhaps the newsletter can best be summed up by a quote from its masthead: "*Natural Living Newsletter* is meant to be one of many sources of information to help people take responsibility for their own health." Rather than present several short articles on different topics, each issue is devoted to a single topic, often to be continued in the following one. Several topics discussed in recent issues have been:

- ▪ Immunity system
- ▪ Losing weight
- ▪ Testing and treating of food allergies
- ▪ Electromagnetic pollution.

Nutrition for Optimal Health Association, Inc.
P.O. Box 380
Winnetka, IL 60093
708-835-5030

▌ Background

Nutrition is something you can do for yourself. It may be the best means of preventing many of the major illnesses we fear will strike us. Whether through vitamin, mineral, or other supplements or through carefully prepared whole foods, nutrition may be the most important thing you can do to assure your own longevity in good health.

What information you need, where to get it, and how to apply it remain open questions to many. Nutrition for Optimal Health

Association (NOHA), Inc. is an educational organization of health care professionals. It provides a diversity of alternative ideas for interested individuals.

▌ What's Offered

If you live in the greater Chicago area, a $25 membership fee will entitle you to admission to NOHA's many events, educational materials, and a subscription to their newsletter. The quarterly ($8), *NOHA News*, is available to nonmembers and is devoted to nutritional news culled from many scientific and lay sources.

NOHA also sells many audio tapes and videos by famous scientists, nutritionists, doctors, and dentists including topics such as:

- Delaying the aging process
- Nutrition and antisocial behavior
- Bioecologic illness—environment/body connection
- Nutrition for immunity
- Reversing diabetes
- Magnesium—cellular health
- Nutrition—academic performance
- Vision and health.

Nutrition Health Review
171 Madison Avenue
New York, NY 10016
212-679-3590

▌ Background

Nutrition Health Review a tabloid-sized, 26-page newsletter published eight times a year ($15), addresses health, disease prevention, and treatment from an alternative treatment perspective but with a vegetarian twist.

▌ What's Offered

This is not yet another publication espousing vegetarianism and crammed with vegetarian recipes, although it does (gently) espouse vegetarianism. Rather, it is a health and medical newsletter.

Although scholarly, well-researched, and literate, I defy you to find jargon or scientific obfuscation. Each issue has a theme: Anxiety, the heart, osteoporosis, and prescription drugs were recently covered. As an example, the issue devoted to wasting diseases had an article on amyotrophic lateral sclerosis (Lou Gehrig's disease), one on muscular dystrophy, and another on multiple sclerosis. Many articles are in a question-and-answer format and discuss prevention and alternative treatments.

Regular columns feature:

- Health and medical news from around the world
- Answers to readers' questions on health and nutrition
- Herbal remedies for readers' health problems
- Natural beauty column
- Book reviews.

Prevention
Rodale Press, Inc.
33 East Minor Street
Emmaus, PA 18098
215-967-5171

▌ Background

Prevention, perhaps America's most famous monthly magazine of alternative health ($15.97), is now perhaps as much mainstream as it is complementary. Nonetheless, the surgical knife and prescription drugs are considered as last resorts, not as knee-jerk, first-and-only treatments.

▌ What's Offered

This full color, near 150-page pocket-sized magazine is available at almost every newsstand and public library. Every article is well researched and usually contains quotes from and references to experts in the field. Most health-related articles include resources (although most are orthodox rather than complementary) for your follow up. Monthly regular columns include medical news and health tips, food and nutrition science research findings, a readers' column, and editorial advice. Before passing judgment on just how alternative the information offered is, sample a few issues. Of the many topics presented in just the past few issues, here are some samples:

- ▌ Health spa menus
- ▌ Milk and cancer
- ▌ Controlling diabetes
- ▌ Aspirin for the heart
- ▌ New arthritis treatments
- ▌ Medical yoga
- ▌ Overcomng shingles pain.

Preventive Medical Update
HealthComm,Inc.
5800 Soundview Drive
#E-102
P.O. Box 1729
Gig Harbor, WA 98335
206-851-3943
206-851-9749 (fax)

▌ Background

The monthly volume of medical and nutritional information published in peer-reviewed journals is enormous. Even health care
professionals and academics cannot keep up.

Preventive Medical Update, a monthly ($199), 90-minute audio
tape magazine, reviews and presents the most important findings
of nutrition.

▌ What's Offered

*Preventive Medical Update'*s regular features include an interview
with an innovative practitioner, a medical news summary, and an
in-depth analysis of the latest research in one topic. Summary
sheets of the articles reviewed and a bibliography accompany the
tape.

HealthComm also publishes several other items of interest.
Focus on Vitality, an eight-page quarterly ($10) on nutrition and its
effects on health, contains short articles on the latest health news
and current medical and scientific research.

Several audio tape courses on nutrition and detoxification are
also offered for sale.

Society of Prospective Medicine
P.O. Box 55110
Indianapolis, IN 46205-0110
317-549-3600   317-549-3670 (fax)
Contact: Pamela Hall, Managing Director

▌ Background

Can you go through life without risks? I doubt it. Can you even arrange your life so that you take no risks to endanger your own health? Again, I doubt it.

What you can do however, is appraise risks that may endanger your health. For example, sunlight is undeniably good for you, but too much can cause skin cancer. Fats are essential to life and health; Without some fat in your diet you would die. But eating a diet of potato chips and hamburgers to get your fat is a poor choice for two reasons. First, the risks imposed by that diet far outweigh any benefits you would receive. Second, there are healthier ways to get both the amount and kind of fat you need in your diet.

The Society of Prospective Medicine (SPM) is concerned with encouraging individuals and organizations to set high standards of health-risk appraisal. Its stated goals are:

- ▌ To extend life expectancy by identifying and reducing health risks
- ▌ To disseminate information about risk reduction
- ▌ To encourage research
- ▌ To promote the teaching of health-risk reduction
- ▌ To assist professionals and groups in implementing health-risk appraisal and reduction programs.

▌ What's Offered

SPM publishes a quarterly ($20) newsletter, *An Ounce of Prevention*, that discusses research in health-risk reduction and lists upcoming events. As a health care consumer, this organization may prove more useful at your place of work than to you as an individual, especially since its thrust is aimed at organizations and professionals.

Proceedings of its conferences are available as well and may serve to help your own company set up a health-risk reduction program of its own.

Spectrum
58 Webster Street
Laconia, NH 03426
603-528-4710

▌ Background

Many respected scientific journals report on topics of importance
to those interested in alternative health care.

Spectrum, a bimonthly ($10), 36-page magazine, reports in
summary form much of the latest research and news from those
journals.

▌ What's Offered

The magazine is divided into eight major sections: food and nutrition, environment, healing, lifestyle, medicine, mind and spirit,
society, and an interview. Each section contains eight to 10 very
short summaries with the name of the scientific journal from which
the information was obtained. Examples of some topics from a
recent issue are:

- PMS and healing with light
- Aloe vera and immunity
- Electromagnetic fields and brain function
- The necessity of breast self-examinations
- Religion and altruism
- Quiet.

Each issue also includes an editorial and a directory of alternative lifestyle and health resources.

Today's Living
Communication Channels, Inc.
6255 Barfield Road
Atlanta, GA 30328
404-256-9800

▌Background

Today's Living is published monthly ($12). A 28-page, full-color magazine, it's usually found at the checkout counters in health food stores; it is often given to customers without charge.

▌What's Offered

Like *Better Nutrition*, its sister publication, *Today's Living*'s articles are jargon-free. Monthly columns include answers to readers' questions, health news, a guide to new products, and a self-test on a health matter. The articles are divided into three broad categories: supplements, body care, and food. They're not at all technical and offer practical advice and case histories rather than theory. All have references to make it easy for you to get more detailed information. Almost anyone should be able to go cover-to-cover in less than an hour and will likely pick up at least a few facts that made the trip worthwhile. Some recent articles have been on:

■ Obesity and diet therapies
■ Zinc for skin problems, metals poisoning, prostate problems, and colds
■ Gum-disease prevention
■ Natural remedies for chronic headaches
■ Oat and rice bran for cholesterol
■ Phosphate detergent ban
■ Low-fat ethnic menus
■ Health benefits of pineapple.

Further Resources
> American College of Nutrition
> American Nutrimedical Association
> *Balance*
> Bio-Research For Global Evolution
> Canadian Schizophrenia Foundation
> *Cardiac Alert*
> Council for Responsible Nutrition
> Heart Disease Research Foundation
> Hippocrates Health Institute
> HOPE Heart Institute
> Huxley Institute for Biosocial Research, Inc.
> *International Journal of Biosocial and Medical Research*
> Life Extension Foundation
> Linus Pauling Institute of Science and Medicine
> Maharishi Ayur-Veda Association of America
> *Natural Healing Newsletter*
> North American Nutrition & Preventive Medicine Foundation, Inc.
> *Nutrition Action Healthletter*
> *Nutrition and Cancer*
> *Nutrition News*
> *Nutrition Report*
> Price-Pottenger Nutrition Foundation
> Princeton BioCenter

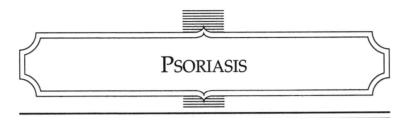

PSORIASIS

National Psoriasis Foundation
6443 SW Beaverton Highway
Suite 210
Portland, OR 97221
503-297-1545
503-292-9341 (fax)

Contact: Glennis McNeal, Public Information Director

▌Background

Psoriasis, often the subject of cruel jokes, is not merely a skin rash. It affects 2% of Americans, or almost four million people. Each year 150,000 new cases occur. Some cases are so bad that orthodox medicine treats them with a form of chemotherapy. Some joke!

Although there are more than two dozen types of psoriasis, they all are chronic skin disorders, appearing as scaly patches. All types of this incurable disease occur when certain skin cells reproduce faster than normal and do not fully mature. Its cause is unknown. All treatments, both orthodox and alternative, help the skin's appearance but do not seem to affect a permanent cure.

The National Psoriasis Foundation (NPF) was founded to encourage research into the causes of and cures for psoriasis, to educate the general public, and to provide information and support for sufferers.

▌What's Offered

Membership in the NPF is open to anyone for any donation. For it you will receive the *Bulletin*, the Foundation's bimonthly newsletter. In it you'll find a readers' query column, members tips for coping, and information on local support groups. Recent articles have covered the following topics:

- Psoriasis and diet
- Psoriasis and the nervous system
- Yeast and microbe complications
- Scales—removing them
- Remedies—tar
- Itching—what you can do
- Nail psoriasis.

The Foundation publishes more than two dozen pamphlets on different types of psoriasis. The pamphlets include explanations, causes, self-help information, and types of professional treatments available. A physician referral service is also available.

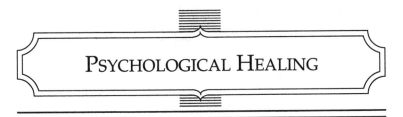

PSYCHOLOGICAL HEALING

American Art Therapy Association, Inc.
1202 Allanson Road
Mundelein, IL 60060
708-949-6064

▌ Background

Psychological counseling and treatment has gone far beyond Freud and Jung, and it finds little use for American behaviorism. One means of counseling is through a patient's art. By watching and analyzing the behavior of a patient making art and the art itself, a trained therapist can often gain insight into that patient's mental state.

The American Art Therapy Association (AATA), Inc., a professional organization of licensed art therapists, is devoted to the therapeutic use of art. Its purpose is:

- ▪ To set standards of clinical practice
- ▪ To provide a network for communication between professionals
- ▪ To promote the field through dissemination of information to the public.

▌ What's Offered

The AATA's official publication ($25), *Art Therapy*, presents case studies, research findings, and clinical research. A quarterly ($16) newsletter relates upcoming events, seminars, and conferences which are held by the AATA. They also publish many books on the profession.

American Association for Music Therapy
P.O. Box 27177
Philadelphia, PA 19118
215-242-4450

Contact: Katie Hartley, Executive Director

▌ Background

Music therapy has successfully been used for mental health ailments, developmental disabilities, Alzheimer's disease, substance abuse problems, brain injuries, physical disabilities, and chronic illness.

Associated with the National Association for Music Therapy (see below), the American Association for Music Therapy (AAMT) is a professional organization of music therapists. It helps establish standards of professional competence and implements them through certification of individuals and university curricula.

▌ What's Offered

Aside from an annual conference, AAMT publishes several journals and sponsors conferences: *Music Therapy*, their premier technical journal, primarily concerns itself with research and therapeutic developments in the field; *Tuning In*, a newsletter, provides a dialogue among music therapists and serves as a forum to discuss treatment modalities; and *Music Therapy International Report* reports on music therapy research from 20 countries.

A membership directory is available to help you find a nearby professional.

American Council of Hypnotist Examiners
312 Riverdale Drive
Glendale, CA 91204
818-242-1159
818-247-9379 (fax)

▌ Background

Hypnosis is neither a deep sleep nor unconsciousness. Rather, it is a unique form of consciousness affecting the left side of the brain. Its chief attribute is extreme suggestibility. When in this hypnotic state of suggestibility, a person will feel no pain when told that the needle sticking through his or her palm does not hurt, and will do the outrageous things he or she wouldn't dream of doing normally when told to do so by the hypnotist.

However, these stage tricks aside, hypnotherapy's use of the hypnotic state is in allowing repressed memories to be released into conscious awareness. It is believed that many psychological problems (and some physiological ailments as well) are the result of repressed thoughts and feelings.

The American Council of Hypnotist Examiners (ACHE) is a non-profit, professional organization that sponsors conferences and seminars, and offers advanced training for practitioners. Through its efforts in establishing professional training centers, ACHE:

▪ Establishes standards for, and certifies hypnotherapists
▪ Provides training and qualifying examinations for hypnotherapists.

ACHE is especially concerned with so-called hypnotists who receive degrees (some which give them the idea that they are "doctors" of hypnotism) in weekend seminars and who then immediately go into practice.

▌What's Offered

While membership is not open to the non-professional, ACHE can help you find a certified hypnotherapist in your area when you write or telephone.

American Dance Therapy Association
2000 Century Plaza
Suite 108
Columbia, MD 21044
301-997-4040

Contact: Stephanie S. Katz

▌Background

Dance—whether the graceful and civilized minuet or whatever passes for dance in today's clubs—has always been viewed as a primal response to rhythm and music. Many cultures attribute magical powers to dance. Nearly all who dance have, at times, felt more in touch with themselves while dancing.

Dance or movement therapy is the psychotherapeutic use of movement. It is primarily used as part of psychotherapy or as a means of assessing the psychological health of an individual. Practitioners must not only be skilled in the art of dance but be thoroughly trained in psychotherapy.

The American Dance Therapy Association (ADTA) is the professional organization of dance therapists. It sets educational standards and sees to the training of its members.

▌What's Offered

The ADTA publishes the *American Journal of Dance Therapy,* many monographs, conference proceedings, and several books on dance therapy. All material is technical and written exclusively for the professional or student.

If you wish further information or a referral to a professional dance therapist in your area, write or telephone.

American Horticultural Therapy Association
9220 Wightman Road
Suite 300
Gaithersburg, MD 20879
301-948-3010

▌ Background

What's the most popular outdoor activity in America? Surprisingly, it's not a sport, but gardening. And, since most home gardeners do not grow food, it's clear that they garden for pleasure. Anyone who has gardened knows the satisfaction of growing things. Several years ago professional health care workers thought of bringing that satisfaction or just bringing plants into the environment of people who are physically or developmentally disabled or mentally ill.

Founded almost 20 years ago; the American Horticultural Therapy Association (AHTA), is the professional organization of horticultural therapists. Its goal is to promote and develop horticultural therapy as a therapeutic and rehabilitative medium.

▌ What's Offered

Membership in the AHTA is open to both professionals and interested individuals. It also publishes the *Journal of Therapeutic Horticulture* annually and a directory of all its members.

Should you wish a referral or need additional information on horticultural therapy, the AHTA will be happy to help you.

American Society of Group Psychotherapy and Psychodrama
6728 Old McLean Village Drive
McLean, VA 22101
703-556-9222

▌ Background

Much of modern psychological counseling takes place in a group setting. People with similar or related problems come together and help each other as much as the professional conducting the treatment session. The notion of group therapy has expanded beyond small groups of patients led by a counselor.

Two methods developed during the 1960s and 1970s are psychodrama and sociometry. Psychodrama utilizes guided dramatic action to examine problems raised in a group therapy setting. Sociometry studies groups: how they form and how people in the group relate to each other.

The American Society of Group Psychotherapy and Psychodrama (ASGPP) is a professional organization of therapists employing psychodrama and utilizing sociometry in their group therapy practice. Like most other professional groups, it:

- ▌ Sets standards of clinical practice
- ▌ Provides a network for communication between professionals
- ▌ Promotes the field through dissemination of information to the public.

▌ What's Offered

The ASGPP publishes the *Journal of Group Psychotherapy, Psychodrama and Sociometry* devoted primarily to articles in experimental research and empirical and clinical studies. Its quarterly newsletter, *Psychodrama Network News*, contains information about upcoming workshops, reviews of books, and other materials.

American Society of Pastoral and Wellness Counselors
P.O. Box 723
Colorado Springs, CO 80901

▌ Background

Long before there were professional psychotherapists, people had psychological problems. What did they do? Often, they talked to a spouse, other relative, or a friend. But some problems were felt to be too embarrassing and couldn't be discussed. Then a person went to someone in the community whose life was service to that community: a priest, pastor, or rabbi.

The American Society of Pastoral and Wellness Counselors (ASP&WC) is a professional organization of holistic-oriented health care practitioners who use pastoral counseling.

▌ What's Offered

Membership is open only to professionals who are licensed and hold degrees in counseling, psychology, theology, or pastoral counseling whose practice is based upon scripture and theology.

A referral to a licensed, professional counselor in your area is available if you write.

Association for Applied Psychophysiology and Biofeedback
10200 West 44th Avenue   Suite 304
Wheat Ridge, CO 80033
303-422-8436   303-422-8894 (fax)

▌ Background

Biofeedback, the rage of the 1960s, allows you to become aware of the body functions that you usually take for granted. After that awareness, biofeedback can train you to use your body's own signals to improve your health. It allows you to have control over what were once thought of as automatic functions beyond human change. It has been successfully used to:

- Relieve migraine and tension headaches
- Lower high blood pressure
- Relieve chronic pain
- Reduce many forms of tension
- Relieve stress-related respiratory problems
- Treat epileptics to control their seizures
- Help stroke victims regain movement in paralyzed muscles.

The Association for Applied Psychophysiology and Biofeedback (AAPB) is an organization of professionals, not of laypersons. Most of its members are biofeedback and applied psychophysiological practitioners. These include psychologists, psychiatrists, physical rehabilitation professionals, dentists, nurses, and educators, many of whom are also on the staff of universities and conduct clinical research.

▌ What's Offered

Aside from professional meetings at which research papers are presented, the AAPB offers its members a subscription to the quarterly *Biofeedback and Self Regulation*, its official publication.

While the proceedings, workshops, and publications are quite technical, recent topics have included:

- Postural distortion
- Emotional self-regulation
- Post-traumatic headaches
- Respiration awareness and breathing
- Biofeedback and stress reduction
- Anxiety disorders
- Psychopharmacology
- Chronic pain therapies.

For those with a technical bent and a desire for further information, workshop proceedings are available in print and on audio tape. Many books and audio tapes on biofeedback can also be ordered from the Association's catalogue.

The Association maintains a list of its more than 2200 members and will help you to find a practitioner in your area.

Association for Humanistic Psychology
1772 Vallejo Street #3
San Francisco, CA 94123
415-346-7929

▌ Background

Help for a psychological problem—even information on psychological issues—is available from a variety of sources. Theories are rampant. Alternative approaches, orthodox treatments, pharmaceuticals, and physical therapies seem to outnumber the persons seeking relief.

The Association for Humanistic Psychology (AHP) is a professional organization of health care practitioners and educators.

▌ What's Offered

Believing that many problems are fostered by the feelings resulting from a lack of attaining one's ultimate potential, humanistic psychology utilizes a variety of psychological and physical therapeutic approaches to relieve symptoms and resolve issues.

As a professional organization, the AHP publishes the quarterly *Journal of Humanistic Psychology*, a technical journal of clinical studies and treatment modalities, and the bimonthly newsletter *AHP Perspectives*, encompassing numerous short articles on the practical applications of different approaches to well-being as well as news of the organization and a calendar of upcoming events.

Membership is open to anyone, and many of the publications and conferences provide information that even nonprofessionals will find of value. But what might prove of most value is a directory of members from which you may find a health care practitioner.

Association for Past-Life Research and Therapies, Inc.
P.O. Box 20151
Riverside, CA 92516
714-784-1570

Contact: Sylvia Alfred

▮ Background

Déjà vu: the feeling that you've been somewhere before, even when you know you've never been there. Many people have experienced it. Past-lives: The feeling that you've lived before. Some people believe they have.

Anyone troubled by the feeling that they have lived before as someone else usually seeks psychological help. A recognized form of therapy is past-life recall or regression therapy.

The purpose of the Association for Past-Life Research and Therapies (APRT), Inc. is to serve as a professional organization and training ground for past-life therapists.

▮ What's Offered

APRT publishes the *APRT Newsletter*, a quarterly ($10) review of articles in regression therapy; upcoming events, conferences, and training programs; book reviews; and members' news. The *Journal of Regression Therapy*, a biannual ($15) professional journal of clinical practice and case histories, is also available by subscription. Recent article topics have included:

- ▮ Imaging techniques in past-life therapy
- ▮ Philosophical assumption of past-life therapy
- ▮ Brain wave states in regression states
- ▮ Hypnosis and healing
- ▮ Karmic view of polio
- ▮ Folk healing traditions.

Referrals for a past-life therapist in your area will be individually handled.

Association for Transpersonal Psychology
P.O. Box 3049
Stanford, CA 94309
415-327-2066

▮ Background

Indeed, "no man is an island" any longer. In one way or another all of us are a part of each other. This is the view of transpersonal psychology—that all life is interconnected.

Professional therapists using a transpersonal approach stress the need to understand the relationships we have both with other people and to everything on the planet.

The Association for Transpersonal Psychology (ATP) is the professional organization of transpersonal psychotherapists. It sets educational standards, helps its memebrs pursue further training, and seeks to disseminate knowledge of psychological inter-connectivity from a transpersonal perspective. This perspective includes:

- Intuition and awareness
- Change and personal transformation
- Spiritual paths and practices
- Self-realization and higher values.

▌ What's Offered

ATP publishes a quarterly newsletter as well as its premier journal, the *Journal of Transpersonal Psychology*, which focuses on objective and subjective transpersonal experiences, concepts, and practices. Although written by professionals for other professionals, laypersons will not find it difficult going. All topics are thoroughly discussed, well-researched, and contain citations. Article topics have included:

- Voluntary control of internal states
- Meditation—EEG biofeedback
- Altered states of consciousnes—scientific validation
- Brain-wave activity—changes during channeling
- Morita therapy.

If you wish further information or a referral to a professional in your area, write or telephone.

National Association for Drama Therapy
19 Edwards Street
New Haven, CT 06511
203-624-2146

■ Background

Drama therapy is the use of drama, theater, and role-playing for emotional and physical rehabilitation.

The National Association for Drama Therapy (NADT) is an accreditation and professional organization.

■ What's Offered

Aside from its professional aspects, the NADT publishes several books, monographs, and audio tapes as well as its newsletter, *Dramascope*. Published twice a year ($5) and available to nonmembers, each issue has articles, book reviews, news and information about upcoming events, and profiles of people in the drama therapy field.

If you have an interest in drama therapy or believe that it may help you or someone you know, contact the NADT, which will answer any questions and help you to locate a professional in your area.

National Association for Music Therapy
505 11th Street, SE
Washington, DC 20003
202-543-6864

■ Background

Music has a powerful, and at times, hypnotic effect upon the body and the mind. It is for this reason—the ability to penetrate below the level of consciousness—that it is used as a therapy.

Music therapy aims to restore mental and physical health through the playing of music under certain stressful conditions.

These include hospitals, clinics, day-care facilities, schools, mental health centers, nursing homes, and so forth.

The National Association for Music Therapy (NAMT) is a professional organization of practitioners who use music as part of their therapeutic approach to psychological disorders.

▋ What's Offered

The NAMT publishes three journals: *Journal of Music Therapy*, a quarterly devoted to original music therapy research; *Music Therapy Perspectives*, an annual monograph on professional practices that can be utilized by other professionals; and *NAMT Notes*, an eight-page, bimonthly newsletter of upcoming events and news of interest to the members.

If you believe that music therapy can help you or a loved one, are a professional who would like further information, or are just an interested individual, the Assocation will provide you with data on membership and its extensive publication list.

National Association for Poetry Therapy
225 Williams Street
Huron, OH 44839
416-433-5018

Contact: George L. Bell

▋ Background

The mind is still a vast uncharted territory. Mapping the brain successfully will only help us get to shallow waters. Many easy-to-understand things may cause psychological problems: diet, disease, allergens, side effects of drugs, lack of essential nutrients. The hard part occurs when there is no underlying physical cause, but where the cause is the mind itself.

One therapeutic modality that has shown promise in problems of the mind is poetry therapy. The National Association for Poetry Therapy (NAPT) is the information source for this practice and serves as an educational center and a certification agency for its practitioners.

▌ What's Offered

Membership is $40. For that you will receive two publications. The monthly 22-page newsletter, the *NAPT Newsletter*, publishes short, newsy tidbits concerning members: members' news and coming events. The quarterly ($32), *Journal of Poetry Therapy*, publishes original articles on the poetic in health.

An available directory of members will allow you to seek a professional in your area.

National Association of Neuro-Linguistic Programming, Inc.
310 North Alabama
Suite A100
Indianapolis, IN 46204
317-636-6059
317-638-0539 (fax)

Contact: Laura S. Shaw

▌ Background

Although we all live in the same world of objective reality, each of us has a subjective experience of it.

Neuro-linguistic programming (NLP) studies this subjective experience using specific means of communicating. The NLP process results in a change in behavior and emotional states. This new behavior is better able to reach an individual's goals. NLP, though, is used for many things other than psychological counseling: sales and marketing are the most famous.

The National Association of Neuro-Linguistic Programming (NANLP), Inc. is an educational organization of professionals from counseling, psychotherapy, law, medicine, sales, and marketing.

▌ What's Offered

Membership ($25) in NANLP is open only to interested individuals with some NLP training. Members receive the membership directory and the *NLP Connection*. This quarterly contains meeting and conference announcements, policies, and members' articles on NLP practices.

Many NLP publications (and popular books), both technical and popular, from which you can gain a better understanding of this discipline are available.

National Therapeutic Recreation Society
Twelfth Floor
3101 Park Center Drive
Alexandria, VA 22302-1593
703-820-4940

▌ Background

For far too many of us, recreation means television. Outside of working, sleeping, and eating, many (perhaps most) Americans only watch televison, calling it their major recreational activity.

Surprise, America! There was a time when recreation meant more physical movement than reaching for a fistful of munchies and a soft drink.

For people with physical disabilities, who are mentally retarded, or who suffer from mental illness, or older adults, physical recreation can often mean the difference between a life as a permanent shut-in or a life of independence and involvement.

The National Therapeutic Recreation Society (NTRS), associated with the National Recreation and Park Association, is a professional organization of physicians, nurses, therapists, and counselors who use recreational therapy as part of their practice.

Numerous studies have shown that recreation as a therapy can improve physical abilities, build self-confidence, promote self-reliance, ease the fears associated with medical procedures or hospitalization, and manage stress.

▌ What's Offered

Aside from the numerous books available on the subject and their quarterly ($30), *Therapeutic Recreation Journal*, NTRS also maintains a membership directory from which you can locate a member in your area if you believe this form of therapy can help you or someone you know.

Proprioceptive Writing Center
39 Deering Street
P.O. Box 8333
Portland, ME 0414
207-772-1847

▌ Background

Almost everyone can talk about their feelings, even if only to themselves. But very few people can write about them. When we write something, it's as if we are making a commitment to be truthful and accurate, even if only to the blank sheet of paper before us.

Proprioception is a term from the field of physiology that means "feelings that originate in the body's interior." Nerves or proprioceptors send information to the brain that help the body orient itself to movement, direction, and position.

The Proprioceptive Writing Center believes that a special kind of writing enhances one's feeling of self-actualization, satisfies the need to translate experience into language, stimulates the capacity to think deeply about emotions, remember and release emotions, and become more self-reflexive.

▌ What's Offered

Proprioceptive writing classes are presented throughout the country in weekend workshops. The Center also conducts seminars in other aspects of psychological healing such as:

- Thinking and feminism
- Erotic imagination
- Writing and movement
- Feminine consciousness
- Mysticism—East and West.

More information and a series of brochures and books on the therapeutic benefits of proprioceptive writing are also available.

Radix Institute
Route 2
P.O. Box 89-A
Suite 102
Sery Place
Granbury, TX 76048
917-326-5670

Background

It is now accepted that many physiological problems can be helped by manipulative techniques: chiropractic, Rolfing, and the Trager method, to name a few. Many of these manipulative techniques base their treatment upon posture. But can the body's structure, posture, and musculature, along with facial expressions, reveal the mind behind it? In other words, what is the relationship between soma and psyche? The belief of William Reich was that the body and the face, along with the eyes, were the keys to the soul. His work is the basis for Radix training.

The Radix Institute serves as a training center for professionals who will use the neo–Reichian Radix method in their professional practice.

What's Offered

The courses are extensive and require several years of work. This method of training and self-examination is used by other psychological modalities including followers of Freud and Jung. Upon graduation, students may then teach and practice the discipline.

Inquiries concerning Radix teachers who may be of help with any problem you or a family member has may be directed to the Institute.

Sounds True Catalogue
735 Walnut Street
Boulder, CO 80302
800-333-9185 ext. 275
303-449-0058
303-449-9226 (fax)

▌ Background

People, as rational beings, of necessity are also self-reflective beings. But we live in times that fail to appreciate introspection, times
that have traded in the heritage of looking inward for communicating with others. Nature abhors a vacuum. So, too, does society.
Felt needs and desires will always be met, often in ways that are
self-destructive. Is it any wonder that people who cannot tolerate
a moment of being alone seek distraction in everything from
television to drugs? Is it any wonder that this is also a time of
overwhelming psychological pain for many of the best and brightest?

Yet that same vacuum is also being filled with people who
are passing on what they have found in their self-reflection.

Sounds True Catalogue, originally a conference recording service, makes available a wide variety of audio cassettes from hundreds of people who offer new ways of looking inward at oneself
and outward at the world.

▌ What's Offered

Unless you are familiar with New Age thinkers or keep up with
professionals on the edge of psychological thought, many of the
names in this catalogue may be unfamiliar to you. Even when a
name or a way of thinking seems familiar, it is often easier to pick
up important highlights by listening to an audio tape than by
reading a book.

Some of the subjects available include:

- Relationships
- Psychology and spirit
- Health and healing
- Meditation
- Life and death
- Conference proceedings.

The catalogue is well prepared, and every entry will give you sufficient information to let you know what you will be getting if you order a tape. Tapes and sets usually run about $10 per 60- or 90-minute cassette.

_____

Further Resources
   see all resources under MIND–BODY CONNECTION
   see all resources under ORTHOMOLECULAR NUTRITION AND
      THERAPY

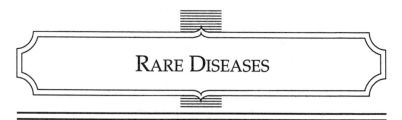

RARE DISEASES

National Organization for Rare Disorders, Inc.
P.O. Box 8923
New Fairfield, CT 06812-1783
800-447-NORD
203-746-6518

Contact: Dr. Jess Thorne, President

▌ Background

The National Organization for Rare Disorders (NORD), Inc. serves as a clearinghouse for information on rare disorders and monitors the federal government's handling of the 1983 Orphan Drug Act. This act encourages pharmaceutical companies to develop and make available drugs and treatments for rare diseases without their having to go through the FDA's time-consuming (three to five years) and costly (upwards of $120 billion) process.

NORD also serves as a coordinating agency for over 100 other organizations exclusively devoted to a single disease: acoustic neuroma to Wilson's disease.

▌ What's Offered

Grants are made available for promising research projects (many of which require an advanced degree to understand), and a quarterly ($25) magazine, *Orphan Disease Update* is published to keep members informed of events. Recent article topics discussed have included:

- ▌ Health insurance—how to obtain coverage

- Orphan Drug Act amendments
- Biomedical research—causes and treatments
- Gene defects
- Small-business health insurance for rare disorders
- Handicapped children
- Toxic shock syndrome
- Readers' mailbox—queries and tips
- Current research.

NORD also has hundreds of inexpensive brochures and pamphlets on nearly 5000 rare diseases. A recent patient workshop discussed coping, dealing with doctors, employment concerns, hospitals, imagery and relaxation, and the family.

Although not primarily concerned with treatments for individual patients, NORD will help you find therapies (alternative or orthodox) for rare diseases and their practitioners.

RESPIRATORY ILLNESSES

**National Jewish Center For Immunology
and Respiratory Medicine**
1400 Jackson Street
Denver, CO 80206-2762
800-222-LUNG

■ Background

Imagine always gasping for air, not being able to breathe freely, or
continually coughing. Imagine not knowing where to get help or
even what it is.

When illness strikes, even when it's only in its infancy, just
knowing what the ailment is called helps. Getting answers to your
questions can be the most helpful thing for you.

The National Jewish Center For Immunology and Respiratory Medicine is recognized as one of the nation's best hospitals
specializing in chronic respiratory diseases. It is also one of the best
sources for information about the 23 lung-related ailments that
range from asthma to vocal chord constriction.

■ What's Offered

The Center maintains a toll-free telephone service called the Lung
Line. It's a free consumer information service, handling thousands
of calls a month on a wide variety of topics related to respiratory
illness. Specially trained nurses answer questions about early diagnosis, care and prevention, treatments, and helping yourself. A
tiny sample of the topics includes:

- Exercise-induced asthma
- Asthma and pregnancy
- Emphysema
- Medications
- Immunological disorders
- Occupational lung diseases.

Packets of literature are sent free to any requester. This information consists of easy-to-read booklets that explain the condition, coping with it, what research offers in the way of treatments, and what therapies are currently available.

Further Resources
    see all resources under ASTHMA

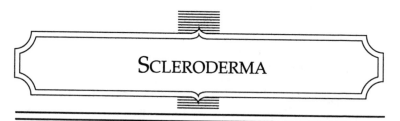

SCLERODERMA

Scleroderma Association
P.O. Box 910
Lynnfield, MA 01940
508-535-6600

▌ Background

Scleroderma, meaning hard skin in Greek, usually affects women of childbearing age. Not limited only to the skin, it often damages the esophagus, intestinal tract, heart, lungs, and kidneys as well; often debilitating its sufferers, occasionally resulting in their death.

The Scleroderma Association is a nonprofit, grass-roots organization of volunteers providing information to patients and their families.

▌ What's Offered

To support itself, the Association publishes a 16-page quarterly ($15), *The Beacon*. Much of the information in this newsletter concerns itself with offering mutual support to fellow sufferers. Other articles discuss new treatments and symptom relief such as:

- ▌ Hydrocolloid membrane treatment for skin ulcers
- ▌ Linear scleroderma patient prognosis
- ▌ Raynaud's disease
- ▌ Over-the-counter and alternative treatments
- ▌ L-tryptophan.

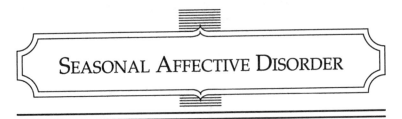

SEASONAL AFFECTIVE DISORDER

Environmental Health & Light Research Institute, Inc.
16057 Tampa Palms Boulevard
Suite 227
Tampa, FL 33647
800-LIGHTS-U

Contact: Fred M. Mendelsohn

▌ Background

Everything on the earth starts with the sun. Every form of energy is ultimately derived from sunlight. Life itself depends on the sun.

The Environmental Health & Light Research Institute (EHLRI), Inc. is committed to studying and conducting research on the relationship between light, radiation, and health. This broad range of subjects includes the beneficial effects of sunlight and full-spectrum artificial light for hyperbillirubinemia, seasonal affective disorder, depression, weight gain, sleep disorders, and pre-menstrual syndrome.

▌ What's Offered

EHLRI was started in 1957 by noted scientist John Ott, who discovered the beneficial effects of full-spectrum light on biological systems. ELHRI sells all of Ott's published work and publishes an eight-page, bimonthly ($29.95) newsletter, *Modern Wellness*. Most issues are devoted to a single subject. An issue is covered in detail: well-researched, practical advice along with theoretical background, filled with resources for following up. For example, a recent issue discussed the harmful effect of low level radiation emitted by video display terminals.

National Organization for Seasonal Affective Disorder
P.O. Box 40133
Washington, DC 20016

▌ Background

We humans, as have all other species on the earth, have evolved under the ever-present sun. Biological rhythms of day and night— circadian rhythms—are understood by laypersons and health professionals alike. Who among us hasn't had an off day?

Less understood are seasonal changes of light and darkness, warmth and cold, plenty and scarcity. Poets, playwrights, and ancient philosophers have long spoken of the affect of seasons: "a sad tale best for Winter" (William Shakespeare). But modern medical orthodoxy, until quite recently, has pooh-poohed the whole notion as un-scientific.

Does your autumn tell of color or the dire threat of the coming winter? Is your winter a time of cozy firesides or a cheerless and foreboding hoary frost? Even spring—a time of blossoming and rebirth—is spoken ill by some: "April is the cruelest month" (T. S. Eliot).

The National Organization for Seasonal Affective Disorder (NOSAD) is a patient support group of sufferers of seasonal affective disorder (SAD).

▌ What's Offered

Membership is open to anyone—patients, friends, family, health care professionals, interested lay people. NOSAD's goals are:

- To disseminate information on SAD to the public and health care professionals
- To provide emotional support and help to SAD sufferers through local support groups
- To act as advocates for SAD patients in the fields of insurance coverage and legislature.

Do you have less energy when the seasons change? Are you sad or even depressed when one season rolls into the next? When the seasons change, do you need more sleep or have problems related to sleep? Do you find that you have no control over your appetite or weight when the seasons change? These or just about any other seasonal-related symptoms might mean you are suffering from SAD.

Current treatment is simple: supplying a source of full spectrum light for an hour or so every day when fall and winter come.

NOSAD, and its quarterly newsletter, offer both information on SAD, emotional support, and help in forming your own local support group if one has not already been started in your area.

Further Resources
  Bio-Electro-Magnetics Institute
  International Journal of Biosocial and Medical Research

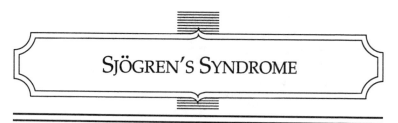

SJÖGREN'S SYNDROME

Sjögren's Syndrome Foundation, Inc.
382 Main Street
Port Washington, NY 11050
516-767-2866

▌ Background

Do you know someone who always has dry eyes, mouth, or nose, often accompanied by arthritis? These are the symptoms of Sjögren's syndrome (SS). SS is a chronic autoimmune disease in which the body's own lymphocytes attack and destroy the exocrine (mucus-secreting) glands. The result is the absence of tears and saliva with accompanying irritation, grittiness, and burning in the eyes and throat.

The Sjögren's Syndrome Foundation's stated purposes are:

- To educate patients and their families and help them to cope
- To increase public and medical awareness of SS
- To stimulate medical research and interest.

▌ What's Offered

Annual membership is $25. For it you will receive membership in a local SS group and a subscription to the monthly newsletter, *The Moisture Seekers*. It contains articles on medical news and treatments, health tips for SS patients, and national organization news. Health information in the past has included:

- Dietary recommendations
- Voice disorders

- Food and inflammatory disorders
- The effectiveness of herbal medicines and acupuncture
- Xerostomia
- Allergy susceptibilities.

Several handbooks and pamphlets are available and the Foundation will help you with a referral to an SS specialist in your area.

SPEECH PROBLEMS

American Speech-Language Hearing Association
10801 Rockville Pike
Rockville, MD 20852
301-897-5700

▋ Background

The American Speech-Language Hearing Association (ASHA) is the professional organization and accrediting agency for speech-language pathologists and audiologists who specialize in communication disorders.

▋ What's Offered

ASHA also sponsors conferences, maintains research findings, publishes 11 technical journals, and offers many books and monographs for professionals. However, it also makes available many pamphlets and booklets for the consumer. Some of the topics covered in them are:

- Stuttering
- Hearing aids
- Hearing loss
- Aphasia
- Tinnitus
- Childhood speech and hearing problems
- Speech and hearing problems in the elderly.

Let's Talk, an eight issue per year ($24) newsletter, contains brief articles summarizing current research in the speech pathology field and work originally presented in the organzization's more technical journals.

A telephone call or letter will get you a referral to several professionals in your area.

National Center for Stuttering
200 East 33rd Street
New York, NY 10016
800-221-2483
212-532-1460

Contact: Lorraine Schneider, Administrative Director

▌ Background

One percent of the population of the United States—2 1/2 million Americans—stutter. When we encounter someone who stutters, it's five times more likely to be a man than a woman, and we sympathize with his difficulty, feel helpless that we can't help him get the words out faster, and usually hold in our tendency to chuckle at the way his face contorts while he desperately struggles to speak coherently.

The National Center for Stuttering believes that stuttering has a physical cause—a spasm of the vocal chords; and that the Center has developed a new therapeutical technique for its cure.

▌ What's Offered

Aside from treatment in its many locations around the country, the Center provides:

- Free information for parents of stutterers and adult stutterers
- Free information for speech professionals regarding training.

Additionally, the Center will help you with a referral to a speech pathologist trained in their method in your area if you write or telephone.

National Stuttering Project
4601 Irving Street
San Francisco, CA 94122-1020
415-566-5324

Contact: John Ahlbach

▌ Background

For over 25 years, annual surveys of people's greatest fears come up with different lists. But in every survey the same fear topped the list: fear of speaking before people. Imagine, more Americans fear to speak before others than fear death. People who stutter fear speaking in almost any situation: to one other person, before a group, but most of all on the telephone.

The National Stuttering Project (NSP), an organization of stutterers, endorses no treatment, although many treatments are available and prove of benefit. Instead, NSP stresses self-help for the stuttering child or adult.

▌ What's Offered

A $30 membership to NSP includes a subscription to the four-page, monthly newsletter *Letting Go*. Its articles include information on the causes of stuttering and inspirational stories of members who have overcome some of their personal problems associated with their stuttering.

Other benefits of joining include a list of over 75 local self-help, support groups in every state, information on a variety of treatments and resource organizations devoted to speech problems and stuttering, and a small catalogue of books, brochures, and audio tapes.

Speech Foundation of America
P.O. Box 11749
Memphis, TN 38111-0749

Contact: Jane Fraser, President

▌ Background

Stuttering is a speech impediment that involves difficulty in talking to other people in person and on the telephone. Primarily affecting males, it often starts in childhood and can lead to other psychological problems such as:

- ▌ Profound shyness—avoidance of speaking to anyone
- ▌ Facial muscle tension
- ▌ Learning disbilities.

The Speech Foundation of America (SFA) provides information on stuttering to the public and the professional. The information particularly emphasizes the latest findings of leading speech pathologists. Aside from therapeutical advice, clinical and practical guidelines on prevention are also provided.

▌ What's Offered

SFA's information for the lay public includes:

- ▌ Parental guide to the stuttering child
- ▌ Self-therapy for the adult stutterer

∎ Guide for the teenage stutterer.

Information for the professional speech therapist on the latest treatments and therapies includes:

∎ Contemporary therapies
∎ Prevention and treatment in children
∎ Clinical guidelines.

While not its primary objective, a free list of referrals to speech pathologists who treat stuttering and other related ailments can be obtained by writing.

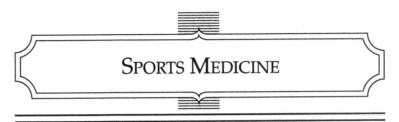

Sports Medicine

American College of Sports Medicine
P.O. Box 1440
Indianapolis, IN 46206-1440
317-637-9200
317-634-7817 (fax)

▋ Background

More people are engaging in recreational sports than ever before.
Unfortunately, an inevitable increase in sports injuries and sports-
related ailments has followed. This has led to the formation of
several sports medicine organizations.

The American College of Sports Medicine (ACSM) does basic
research and disseminates its results and other information on the
benefits and effects of exercise and the treatment and prevention
of injuries incurred in sports, exercise, and fitness programs.

▋ What's Offered

Anyone interested in sports medicine may join the ACSM. Joining
as a non-professional or student will entitle you to receive their
membership directory and the *Sports Medicine Bulletin*, a quarterly
newsmagazine of ACSM's activities, chapter meetings, sports
medicine conferences and meetings, book reviews, and several
special features relating to sports medicine.

Other, more technical publications on sports injuries, their
treatment, and the benefits of different types of exercise are also
available.

While referrals are not directly given, the membership directory (which can be purchased separately) should help you find a professional specializing in sports medicine in your area.

Further Resources
see all resources under PAIN RELIEF

STRESS REDUCTION

American Institute of Stress
124 Park Avenue
Yonkers, NY 10703
914-963-1200

▌ Background

That stress is harmful and that stress can kill and does kill are no longer subjects for debate. It is currently estimated that between 70% and 80% of all visits to a physician are for stress-related disorders. Stress is called the disease of civilization, and stress reduction may be mandatory for a longer, healthier, and more balanced life.

But stress means different things to different people, even professionals. Some basic questions about stress still remain unanswered: Is all stress bad? How much and what kind of stress is harmful? What can be done to reduce stress? What causes stress?

The American Institute of Stress (AIS) was formed as an organization of health care professionals who need timely information on stress.

▌ What's Offered

Membership is open only to professionals. However, two services of the AIS may prove of use to consumers. The first is the eight-page, monthly ($35) *Newsletter of the American Institute of Stress* that contains summaries of articles from other publications, both technical for health professionals, and general for the layperson. Some recent topics have included:

- Electronic brain energizers to relieve stress
- Meditation tapes
- Electrotherapy—stress, addiction
- Foods—heart attacks
- Hostility—type A and coronary heart disease
- Sick buildings—job stress
- Stress reduction—cancer
- Prenatal stress
- Stress and herpes
- Handling stress at work
- Salt—stress and hypertension.

AIS also maintains files, under separate topic headings, of reprints of articles on stress-related subjects from scientific and consumer publications, trade journals, and news media transcripts. Headings range from AIDS to kinesiology, from pregnancy to visual imagery. Lists of titles are available to anyone and may help you to do your own research on a particular stress-related matter.

Flotation Tank Association
P.O. Box 1396
Grass Valley, CA 95945-1396
916-432-3794

Contact: Lee Perry

▌ Background

University research led to the development of flotation tanks. Flotation involves floating in the water of a special tank. When floating, external sensory input is diminished. This places you in a physically relaxed state. In this state, your mind enters a state of consciousness similar to the mental state attained by mystics.

Flotation is used by physicians, psychologists, physical therapists, psychotherapists, chiropractors, and other practitioners as an adjunct to their own treatment. Recent medical findings suggest that flotation can have physical benefits in several chronic diseases.

The Flotation Tank Association, rather than a professional or scientific organization, is a trade association serving to promote the use of flotation for relaxation and to educating the public to its benefits.

▌ What's Offered

A $25 membership fee will get you a subscription to *Floating* and a directory of flotation centers. The magazine has articles on personal experiences of flotation, technical discussions, and news from around the world. Periodic conferences are held on flotation and often discuss the medical and healing applications of flotation.

Article reprints, a bibliography of research papers, audio tapes and videos of past conferences, and several books are also offered.

Myotherapy Institute of Utah
3018 East 3300 South
Salt Lake City, Utah 84109
800-338-8950
801-484-7624
801-467-4792 (fax)

▌ Background

While it is quite common to use massage therapy for muscle pain relief, one of the best results of a massage is the intense feeling of relaxation that one has. In fact, many people use massage therapy solely to relieve stress.

The Myotherapy Institute of Utah is an in-class and home-study school of massage.

▌ What's Offered

The Institute offers classes in such stress relief massage therapies as:

- Spinal touch—light spinal touch
- Magnetic deficiency acupressure—magnets and acupuncture points
- Cranial techniques—osteopathy and cranial rhythms
- Electrostimulation—medium frequency interferential methods
- Tuina acupressure—acupuncture stimulation to release pain
- Basham positional release—relaxing the muscles around a joint
- Reflex activator—reflex gun-stimulation of tonification points.

Many of these techniques are taught in a home-study setting with the use of videos and audio tapes.

The Institute is associated with the Intra-Myomassethics Forum, a professional organization of massage therapists that seeks national certification of the profession.

The Institute will be happy to provide you with a referral to a massage therapist in your area when you telephone their national headquarters at 800-338-8950.

Further Resources
Association for Applied Psychophysiology and Biofeedback
Internal Arts Magazine
Shen Systems
T'ai Chi
Yoga Journal

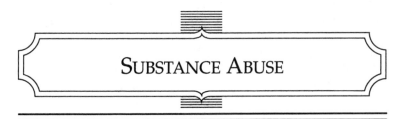

SUBSTANCE ABUSE

Do It Now Foundation
6423 South Ash Avenue
Tempe, AZ 85285
602-491-0393
602-491-2849 (fax)

▋ Background

From the bombardment of information about drug abuse one would think that everybody is snorting cocaine, using crack, smoking marijuana, or injecting themselves with heroin. While clearly not the case, enough people are involved with what is euphemistically called recreational drugs that a political war against them exists at every government and public health level.

The Do It Now (DIN) Foundation was formed 20 years before the war on drugs was declared. DIN believes that everyone is fully responsible for his or her own life and choices about drugs and addiction. Prevention and treatment are best made with the use of accurate and timely information in a context of action rather than as a recital of facts and statistics.

▋ What's Offered

Education on both illegal drugs and the misuse of legal ones is provided through a series of low-cost pamphlets, reports, in-depth current scientific literature and research bibliographies, booklets, and books. Some current topics covered are:

▪ Cocaine

- Marijuana—medical uses, health, personality and behavior problems
- Aspirin
- Valium and Librium—depression
- Alcohol—nutrition, health, interaction with drugs
- Eating disorders
- Anabolic steroids
- Legal stimulants.

Just Say No, International
1777 North California Boulevard
Suite 210
Walnut Creek, CA 94956
800-258-2766
415-939-6666
415-933-8279 (fax)

Background

Opinion polls show that more people are worried about drugs in America than almost anything else. A war on drugs has been declared by every recent President and has been endorsed by every politician. Millions of dollars have been spent on a series of wars with little positive result.

Often, an obvious answer to a problem is overlooked because of its very obviousness. Instead of concentrating exclusively on the source of drugs and the people who sell them, why not concentrate on the people who want them, especially children?

Just Say No (JSN), International's focus is to create a drug-free generation by educating children to the dangers of drugs and helping them to avoid the social pressures involved in choosing not to take something merely because everyone else is. To achieve their goals, four related programs are offered:

- Helping children to avoid peer pressure
- Providing education through clubs and family members
- Promoting recreational activities for group support
- Through a series of service projects such as latchkey programs, helping the hospitalized and homebound sick, and developing community activities for children.

What's Offered

JSN's self-help approach is reinforced with two newsletters: *Just Say Notes*, a sprightly quarterly of upcoming activities, and *Just Say No Newsletter*, a tabloid-sized, quarterly addressed to parents, teachers, and community leaders.

Extensive planning guides for communities, a national network of Just Say No clubs for children aged seven to 14, and several books and pamphlets, complete the program.

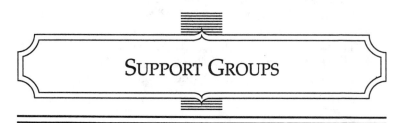

SUPPORT GROUPS

Co-Dependents Anonymous
P.O. Box 33577
Phoenix, AZ 85067-3577
602-277-7991

▌ Background

The poet John Donne aptly said that "no man is an island." That does not mean that we are completely dependent on others. But instead of striking a balance, more people than ever seem to be becoming dependent on someone else for their own identity. This makes the relationship co-dependent.

Co-dependent individuals suffer from:

- ▪ Patterns of denial
- ▪ Low self-esteem
- ▪ Compliance with the wants of others with little regard for themselves
- ▪ Failure to take control of their lives on even the most basic level.

Co-Dependents Anonymous (CoDA) was formed to help those persons who want to form healthy relationships. Loosely modeled after other self-help "anonymous-type" groups, CoDA meetings are highly structured.

▌ What's Offered

CoDA will send you a packet of information that will tell you how to join or start a group and what you can expect from the group sessions.

Several books, audio tapes, and pamphlets are available to help you become better acquainted with the underlying philosophy behind co-dependency and the approaches to helping those suffering from it.

Exceptional Cancer Patients
1302 Chapel Street
New Haven, CT 06511
203-865-8392
203-497-9393 (fax)

▌ Background

What do you believe you would do if you found out that you or one of your family had a life-threatening illness? We all want to believe that we would be calm, act rationally, and search for a therapy that would help. However, when it happens, fear—paralyzing, brain-numbing, panic—often takes over and we are not calm. We do not act rationally, and we fail to search for a helpful therapy. Instead, we run blindly to a physician, crying, "Doctor, you've gotta help me."

Often, the physician can do very little. The therapies work marginally at best. The pharmaceuticals relieve pain but often drug one into insensibility until the end. Many people feel that that's not enough.

Exceptional Cancer Patients (ECP) was founded as an adjunct to orthodox medical therapies: offering psychological support to patients. It has since expanded to include weekly group psychological counseling sessions.

▌ What's Offered

If you would like a referral to a group near you that offers emotional support to sufferers of chronic and life-threatening diseases, or want to help start one, contact ECP.

Also available is a catalogue of books, audio tapes, and videos. It includes information on the psychological aspects of disease and maintaining health.

National Self-Help Clearinghouse
25 West 43rd Street
Room 620
New York, NY 10036
212-642-2944

▌ Background

There are currently an estimated 500,000 self-help groups nationwide. Members are both the helper and the one being helped. The ideas behind self-help groups is that shared problems and feelings make one:

- Feel less isolated when he or she knows that others have the same problem
- Comfortably exchange ideas about handling problems with others who have the same condition
- Gain self-control and make positive lifestyle changes.

The National Self-Help Clearinghouse helps people find a self-help group or organize one in their locality.

▋ What's Offered

There are no membership fees, but several publications are available. The quarterly ($10) *Self-Help Reporter* contains articles on research, advocacy, training, and public policy as they relate to self-help.

Two books on organizing a group can be purchased, and a list of local clearinghouses throughout the United States can be obtained. Enclose a self-addressed, stamped envelope.

State self-help groups maintain a database of all the groups within the state, provide consultation to new groups, publish their own newsletters, provide information and referral to people seeking groups, and publish and sell a variety of material.

Groups normally fall under five broad categories:

- ▪ Addiction and compulsion
- ▪ Bereavement and loss
- ▪ Disabilities
- ▪ Physical and mental health
- ▪ Parenting and family.

Volunteer—The National Center
111 North 19th Sreet
Suite 500
Arlington, VA 22209
703-276-0542
703-528-6021 (fax)

Contact: Kay Drake, Director of Information Services

▋ Background

Have you ever wondered how to contact a local volunteer group in your area for a problem you have? Have you ever wondered if there even is one or how to start one if there is not?

That's the purpose of Volunteer, to help:

■ People become involved in volunteering
■ Develop strong local volunteer groups
■ Increase public awareness, understanding, and the importance of volunteerism
■ Show different ways to apply volunteering to specific problems.

■ What's Offered

If you want to volunteer for something and there's a group that you can join, Volunteer will find it for you. If there isn't, they'll help you to start one. In almost every county of every state, Volunteer has established a "Volunteer Action Center." When you write or telephone, a list of those in your state will be sent to you. Contact the ones closest to you, and they will try to match your needs with a local group.

Voluntary Action Leadership, a quarterly ($20) magazine focuses on the how-to of volunteering with regular legislation columns, tips on personal communicating, book reviews, workshop and conference calendar, articles, and a resource list of inexpensive material.

If you find that there is no group and you want to start one, send $3 for their special "Getting Started in Volunteerism" packet.

Further Resources
International Association of Cancer Victors and Friends, Inc.
Overeaters Anonymous
Patient Advocates for Advanced Cancer Treatments, Inc.

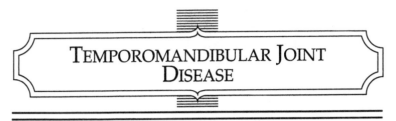

TEMPOROMANDIBULAR JOINT DISEASE

Temporomandibular Joint Research Foundation
3043 Foothill Boulevard
Suite 8
La Crescenta, CA 91214
818-248-9767

Contact: Douglas H. Morgan

∎ Background

Temporomandibular joint (TMJ) disorder affects the hinge of the jaw and the temporal lobes. A person afflicted with TMJ almost always suffers chronic and extreme jaw or dental pain. This is usually the result of jaw misalignment, causing stress. However, many people may feel little or no discomfort and still suffer from TMJ.

The Temporomandibular Joint Research Foundation is concerned with:

- ∎ Teaching health care professionals about treatment approaches
- ∎ Educating the public about TMJ
- ∎ Conducting independent research in TMJ.

∎ What's Offered

Membership in this professional organization is open to dentists and doctors engaged in treating TMJ or researching its cause and cure. Individuals suffering from TMJ may join ($50) one of their support groups (or help establish one) and receive the

Foundation's newsletters. *The TMJ Newsletter* will keep you abreast of the latest developments in the field and informed of which physicians and dentists specialize in TMJ patients. A recently sponsored conference for the medical and dental professions addressed the disease and its treatment. Some topics discussed included:

- TMJ and tinnitus
- Acute muscle spasm treatment
- Surgical alternatives
- Diagnosis
- Chronic facial pain.

Further Resources
American Tinnitus Association

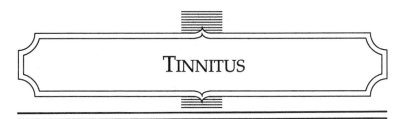

TINNITUS

American Tinnitus Association
P.O. Box 5
Portland, OR 97207
503-248-9985

▌ Background

Tinnitus is ringing in the ear; not the normal and occasional ringing that everyone gets, but continuous and painful ringing. Presently, the cause is unknown and no cure exists.

The American Tinnitus Association (ATA) is a national organization of self-help groups devoted to providing support for tinnitus sufferers.

▌ What's Offered

Joining ATA costs $15. For that you will be put in touch with a local group in your area or assisted in starting one. A quarterly magazine, *Tinnitus Today*, has timely articles on important research and medical news, coping with tinnitus, and causes of tinnitus.

A voluminous bibliography of more than 1800 writings on tinnitus is also available from the ATA. There you will not only learn much about tinnitus but also a great deal about its possible causes such as: drugs, noise, electrical stimulation, smoking, Meniere's disease, trauma, biofeedback, and TMJ.

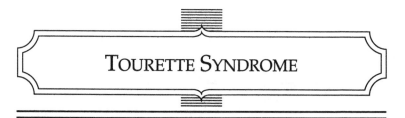

TOURETTE SYNDROME

Tourette Syndrome Association, Inc.
42-40 Bell Boulevard
Bayside, NY 11361-2857
800-237-0717
718-224-2999

Contact: Sue L. Levi

▌ Background

An inherited, neurological disorder characterized by involuntary, rapid, sudden, jerky movements that repeat themselves, Tourette Syndrome (TS) symptoms usually appear before the age of 21. Persons with TS often suffer from:

- Obsessive-compulsive traits
- Hyperactivity
- Attention deficit syndrome
- Learning disabilities
- Sleep disorders.

The Tourette Syndrome Association (TSA), Inc. provides educational information to TS sufferers and their families; helps families cope with problems; and stimulates and supports research into better treatments, the cause, and cure for TS.

▌ What's Offered

Membership dues for TSA are $35. For that you will receive the quarterly, *TSA Newsletter*, with articles on medical news and personal stories of how TS sufferers have successfully coped. Other membership benefits include a discount pharmacy and a discounted registration for conferences.

Much of the educational material offered is quite technical, but very helpful. Reprints of scientific and medical journals constitute the bulk of the newsletter. There are also many brochures and pamphlets suitable for patients and their family members.

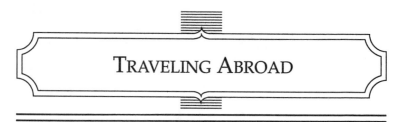

TRAVELING ABROAD

International Association for Medical Assistance to Travelers
447 Center Street
Lewiston, NY 14092
716-754-4883

▌ Background

It's always bad to be sick. But imagine being ill in a foreign country. You can't speak the language. You don't know where to go or whom to see. You feel somewhat like Blanche DuBois—forced to accept the kindness of strangers.

The International Association for Medical Assistance to Travelers (IAMAT) provides travelers with medical information they will find useful when in another country.

▌ What's Offered

Membership in, as well as the services and publications of, the IAMAT is open to any traveler. When you write or telephone, your mailbox will soon contain a thick packet of documents: a directory of English-speaking physicians with a set fee schedule, a series of detailed charts on immunization requirements, information on malaria and other tropical diseases, and climatic and sanitary conditions around the world. If you find the information helpful and useful, a contribution would be appreciated.

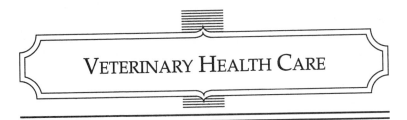

VETERINARY HEALTH CARE

American Holistic Veterinary Medical Association
2214 Old Emmorton Road
Bel Air, MD 21014
301-638-0385
301-638-0385 (FAX)

Contact: Mary Moulsdale

▌ Background

Many families and individuals have pets whom they love. Many of them wish to make sure that those pets receive not only the best of medical care, but also holistic care and alternative treatments to orthodox veterinary care. Until recently, that was difficult to come by. Only if you were fortunate enough to run across a veterinarian open to alternative therapies could you find one.

For that reason, a group of holistic veterinarians was formed. The American Holistic Veterinary Medical Association (AHVMA), is a professional organization of veterinarians devoted to exploring all nonorthodox aspects of veterinary medicine except acupuncture.

▌ What's Offered

Membership in the AHVMA is open only to licensed or student veterinarians and includes a subscription to the Association's quarterly, *Journal of the American Holistic Veterinary Medical Association*. As part of furthering its members' education, it presents technical articles on homeopathy for pets, natural animal nutrients, chronic disease treatments, and vaccine safety and efficacy from a holistic practitioner's viewpoint.

Referrals to a practicing holistic veterinarian in your area are avaialble by telephoning, writing, or faxing the AHVMA.

International Veterinary Acupuncture Society
2140 Conestoga Road
Chester Springs, PA 19425
215-827-7742
Contact: Meredith L. Snader, V.M.D.

∎ Background

That acupuncture is a boon to health care can no longer be disputed by even the most stalwart opponent of complementary medicine. However, it also has a unique place in treating animals. For pets, farm animals, and show animals, acupuncture's primary purpose is to stimulate and strengthen an animal's adaptive/homeostatis mechanism. This is believed to complement their normal defense mechanism and aid in fighting illness and injury.

The International Veterinary Acupuncture Society's purpose is to promote the use of acupuncture in animal care and integrate it into Western veterinary science. It also seeks to bring acupuncture and other overlooked health systems such as homeopathy, herbology, nutrition, chiropractic, kinesiology, and so on into veterinary education.

∎ What's Offered

A newsletter for practitioners, *Veterinary Acupuncture Newsletter*, is available to members, as well as the proceedings of past technical conferences.

Most important to you as a consumer is that you can get a veterinary acupuncturist for your pet. Write to the Society for a list for your state (please enclose $1 to defray costs).

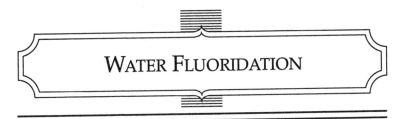

WATER FLUORIDATION

Center for Health Action
P.O. Box 270
Springfield, MA 01138
800-869-9610 (hotline)
413-782-2115

▌ Background

Fluoride, usually in the form of hydrofluosilicic acid, is routinely added to the drinking water of many communities to cut down on dental cavities in children.

But does it? *Nature* magazine of July 10, 1986 reported, after examining flururidation in the United States, that reduction in tooth decay "cannot be attributed to fluoridation. It is time now for a scientific re-examination of the alleged enormous benefits of fluoridation." Fluoride, in the one part per million added to a community's drinking water, is touted as harmless in those quantities. But is it? Studies show that 28% of all children in fluoridated areas develop fluorosis, the first visible sign of permanent and irreversible fluoride poisoning.

The Center for Health Action is opposed to mandatory water fluoridation.

▌ What's Offered

The Center publishes a periodic newsletter, *Update*, reporting on the health risks associated with fluoridation and serves as a national clearinghouse for information on the adverse affects of fluoride in any form, including toothpastes, cavity prevention treatments, and so on.

Safe Water Foundation
6439 Taggart Road
Delaware, OH 43015
614-548-5340

▌ Background

Many American communities add fluoride to their drinking water
in the name of reducing cavities in children. However, there are
many people, including reputable scientists, who believe that fluoridated water poses a profound health risk. They point with
trepidation at several studies linking genetic damage and increased cancer rates to water fluoridation.

The Safe Water Foundation believes that compulsory water
fluoridation poses a significant health risk with no benefit from a
decrease in cavities among children.

▌ What's Offered

The Foundation offers an impressive and long list of clinical studies
to support its case in its fight to preserve fluoride-free water. It also
warns against the use of fluoride treatments, toothpastes, mouth
rinses, tablets, and foods containing fluoridated water.

To support its efforts it sells several books and a variety of
pamphlets on the issue.

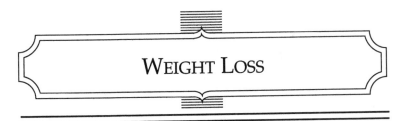

WEIGHT LOSS

Overeaters Anonymous
4025 Spencer Street
Suite 203
Torrance, CA 90503
213-542-8363
213-371-8943 (fax)

Contact: Annette Mambuca

▌ Background

While most people eat too much, all too often many are also compulsive overeaters. A compulsion to eat too much is much like one to drink too much. Diets don't work. Diet clubs don't work. Special diet meals don't work.

Overeaters Anonymous (OA), modeled after Alcoholics Anonymous, is an organization of people who have tried everything else to stop overeating and failed. Much like Alcoholics Anonymous, OA believes in the concept of abstinence. OA members admit their inability to control compulsive eating and forget about eating normally. Instead, OA relies on the idea that you will just not overeat today—just today.

▌ What's Offered

There are no membership dues or membership lists kept; attendees at meeting "pass the hat" to raise funds to hold more meetings.

OA clubs are all over. If you have trouble finding one in your area or wish to start one, contact Overeaters Anonymous for assistance.

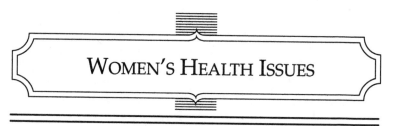

Women's Health Issues

Cesareans/Support Education and Concern
22 Forest Road
Framingham, MA 01701
508-877-8266

█ Background

When a doctor tells a woman that she needs to have a cesarean birth, she almost always will. And that is happening at an alarming rate. Yet it is clear that giving birth is not a new medical procedure. It is equally clear that many other countries have nowhere near the rate of cesarean births that we do in the United States.

The myths surrounding cesareans are as bad as the numbers. How many cesareans can a woman safely have? Can a woman have a normal vaginal birth after cesareans? If a woman has herpes must she have a cesarean?

Cesareans/Support Education and Concern (C/SEC), a non-profit, grass-roots group was formed to help mothers who have undergone cesareans or are considering one. Their goals are:

- █ To provide emotional support for cesarean birth family members
- █ To share information and promote education on cesarean birth, prevention, and vaginal birth after cesarean
- █ To change attitudes and policies affecting cesarean child-birth.

▮ What's Offered

C/SEC publishes a quarterly newsletter, *C/SEC* (all back issues are $2 each). It discusses cesarean prevention and recovery, vaginal birth after cesarean, birth planning, problems arising from herpes, and legal and political issues. Each issue also has several personal experiences from women who have had cesarean births. Topics from back issues include:

- ▮ Midwives' perspective on cesarean
- ▮ Cesarean prevention and recovery
- ▮ Unnecessary cesareans
- ▮ Postpartum depression
- ▮ Fetal distress and monitoring
- ▮ Breech delivery
- ▮ Rise in cesareans and malpractice.

C/SEC also sells several pamphlets and books on cesareans, birthing, and postpartum depression. They will also answer any questions you may have and will help you locate a support group (or start one) in your area.

HERS Foundation
422 Bryn Mawr Avenue
Bala Cynwyd, PA 19004
215-667-7757

▮ Background

More than half the women in the United States will undergo the most commonly performed major surgery. Done at the rate of close to one million procedures yearly, that operation is called a hysterectomy. It has been routinely performed on more than 35 million women; most of them in their mid-30s. It is often accompanied by profound physical and emotional changes.

Slightly more than half a million women have their ovaries removed yearly. If this were done to men, it would be known by its more common name: castration.

Long-term consequences and increased health risks of hysterectomy and female castration include:

- Osteoporosis
- Increased risk of heart disease
- Bone and joint pain
- Loss of sexual desire
- Incontinence
- Emotional changes and depression.

The HERS Foundation, a grass-roots advocacy organization, disseminates information on these subjects.

What's Offered

The Foundation publishes a six-page, quarterly ($20) newsletter, *HERS Newsletter*. It usually includes scientific literature and book reviews, as well as several major articles and letters to the editor. Past issue topics have covered:

- Mental symptoms—effect of estrogen and vitamin B_1
- Sexual response—coping
- Post-hysterectomy syndrome
- Risks—physical and emotional side-effects
- Alternative therapies
- Osteoporosis.

The HERS Foundation also offers publications on the physical and psychological consequences of hysterectomies, alternatives to the operation, and proceedings of many conferences and seminars on the subject.

Other services include helping to form local support groups and free telephone counseling.

Melpomene Institute for Women's Health Research
1010 University Avenue
St. Paul, MN 55104
612-642-1951

▌ Background

Although women constitute more than half the population, most research in health and disease has focused on men. Women's health issues have been discovered only recently.

The Melpomene Institute for Women's Health Research is a center for research on the health concerns of physically active women and the effects of exercise on them.

▌ What's Offered

Annual membership ($25) to Melpomene includes a subscription to the *Melpomene Journal*, published three times a year. Articles have covered such topics as:

- Exercise and menstrual changes—physically active women and girls
- Body image
- Menopause—physical changes, symptoms
- Osteoporosis—prevention, treatment options
- Eating disorders
- Children—socializtion in sports
- PMS—issues, treatments.

Information on women's health issues, in the form of article reprints and brochures, is also available, as well as a video on osteoporosis.

National Women's Health Network
1325 G Street, NW
Washington, DC 20005
202-347-1140

▌Background

Only now is women's health even seen as an issue. While it seems obvious to anyone caring to think about it that women have different health problems from men, almost no one cared to think about it.

The National Women's Health Network, an educational organization, was formed to address women's health matters such as:

- Drugs and medical devices
- Menopause and "replacement" therapy drugs
- Reproductive rights—abortion
- AIDS
- Breast health and cancer
- Maternal and children's health
- Occupational health.

▌What's Offered

Acting as a national clearinghouse for women's health information rather than as a referral service to help you find a health care professional, you may order over 43 separate health information packets on a wide variety of women's health issues. Many books on specific health concerns are available as well.

Women for Sobriety
P.O. Box 618
Quakertown, PA 18951
215-536-8026
Contact: Dr. Jean Kirkpatrick

▌ Background

Alcoholism, once thought to be the province of men, affects women as well. The reasons for it may be unique to women, but it is now a leading health problem among women.

Women for Sobriety believes in a self-help, six-step program only for women consisting of:

▪ Accepting alcoholism as a physical disease
▪ Discarding negative thoughts and feelings
▪ Creating and practicing a new self-image
▪ Fostering new attitudes to change behavior
▪ Improving relationships
▪ Recognizing life's priorities—emotional and spiritual growth.

▌ What's Offered

The Women for Sobriety program is offered free of cost. A self-addressed, stamped envelope will get information to anyone interested.

Further information about the program; their monthly ($15) newsletter, *Sobering Thoughts;* and the many books, workbooks, audio tapes, and videos WFS publishes may also prove of help.

Further Resources
    see all resources listed under CANDIDA ALBICANS
    see all resources listed under CHRONIC FATIGUE SYNDROME
    see all resources listed under EATING DISORDERS
    Endometriosis Association
    National Osteoporosis Foundation
    Overeaters Anonymous
    Scleroderma Association

INDEX

Academy for Guided Imagery, 211-212

Academy of Scientific Hypnotherapy, 202-203

Acupressure Institute of America, 328

AIDS, 1-4

AIDS Treatment News, 1-2

Albert Roy Davis Research Laboratory, 47

Allergic Athlete's Handbook, 5-6

ALLERGIES, 5-9

Allergy Alert, 152

Allergy Information Association, 6-7

Alliance for Aging Research, 228

Alliance for the Prudent Use of Antibiotics, 29-30

Alliance/Foundation for Alternative Medicine, 10-11

ALTERNATIVE HEALING, 10-23

Alternatives For The Health Conscious Individual, 386-387

Alzheimer's Association, 24-25

ALZHEIMER'S DISEASE, 24-26

American Academy of Environmental Medicine, 7-8

American Academy of Husband-Coached Childbirth, 71-72

American Academy of Medical Acupuncture, 329

American Academy of Medical Hypnoanalysts, 203

American Academy of Osteopathy, 353-354

American Aging Association, 229

American Anorexia/Bulimia Association, Inc., 118

American Apitherapy Society, Inc., 46

American Aromatherapy Association, 31-32

American Art Therapy Association, Inc., 421

American Association for Music Therapy, 422

American Association for Therapeutic Humor, 258-259

American Association of Naturopathic Physicians, 290-291

American Association of Orthopaedic Medicine, 354-355

American Board of Chelation Therapy, 68

American Board of Nutrition, 295

American Botanical Council, 184-185

American Celiac Society, 153

American Chiropractic Association, 355-356

American College of Advancement in Medicine, 69-70

American College of Nurse-Midwives, 72-73

American College of Nutrition, 296

American College of Preventive Medicine, 387-388

American College of Sports Medicine, 457-458

American Council for Health Education, 162-163

American Council of Hypnotist Examiners, 423-424

American Dance Therapy Association, 424-425

American Environmental Health Foundation, 126-127

American Federation for Aging Research, Inc., 230

American Foundation of Traditional Chinese Medicine, 330

American Guild of Hypnotherapists, 204

American Health Assistance Foundation, 25-26

American Health Federation, 388-389

American Herb Association, 185-186

American Holistic Medical Association, 11-12

American Holistic Nurses' Association, 12-13

American Holistic Veterinary Medical Association, 477-478

American Horticultural Therapy Association, 425

American Imagery Institute, 212-213

American Institute for Cancer Research, 51-52

American Institute of Biomedical Climatology, 127-128

American Institute of Nutrition, 297

American Institute of Stress, 459-460

American Journal of Clinical Nutrition, 297-298

American Journal of Health Promotion, 219-220

American Longevity Association, 230-231

American Massage Therapy Association, 356-357

American Naprapathic Association, 357-358

American Natural Hygiene Society, 285

American Nutrimedical Association, 298-299

American Nutritionists' Association, 299-300

American Osteopathic Association, 358-359

American Raum & Zeit, 13-14

American Running & Fitness Association, 147-148

Americans for Safe Food, 381

American Social Health Association, 192-193

American Society of Clinical Hypnosis, 205

American Society of Group Psychotherapy and Psychodrama, 426

American Society of Pastoral and Wellness Counselors, 427

American Speech-Language Hearing Association, 452-453

American Sudden Infant Death Syndrome Institute, 88-89

American Tinnitus Association, 473

American Vegan Society, 300-301

AMYTROPHIC LATERAL SCLEROSIS, 27-28

Amytrophic Lateral Sclerosis Association, 27-28

Anorexia Nervosa and Related Eating Disorders, Inc., 119-120

ANTIBIOTICS, 29-30

Archaeus Project, 259-260

Arlin J. Brown Information Center, Inc., 52-53

AROMATHERAPY, 31-34

ARTHRITIS AND OTHER RHEU-MATOID DISEASES, 35-36

ASPO/Lamaze, 73-74

Associated Professional Massage Therapists & Bodyworkers, 359-360

Association for Applied Psychophysiology and Biofeedback, 427-429

Association for Childbirth At Home, International, 74-75

Association for Humanistic Psychology, 429-430

Association for Past-Life Research and Therapies, Inc., 430-431

Association for Research & Enlightenment, Inc., 260-261

Association for Transpersonal Psychology, 431-432

Association of Birth Defect Children, Inc., 89-90

Association of Concerned Citizens for Preventive Medicine, 246

Association of Health Practitioners, 14-15

Association of Holistic Healing Centers, 167-168

ASTHMA, 37-39

Aston-Patterning, 360-361

Aurora Book Companions, 169-170

Australian Wellbeing, 261-262

AUTISM, 40-43

Autism Research Institute, 40-41

Autism Services Center, 41-42

Autism Society of America, 42-43

AYURVEDIC MEDICINE, 44-45

Balance, 220

BEE VENOM THERAPY, 46

Bestways, 389-390

Better Nutrition for Today's Living, 390-391

Bio-Electro-Magnetics Institute, 48-49

Biokinesiology Institute, 279-280

Biological Therapy, 194-195

BIOMAGNETICS, 47-50

Bionomics Health Research Institute, 286

Bio-Research For Global Evolution, 15-16

Bio-Zoe, Inc., 142

Brain/Mind Bulletin, 262-263

Bulimia Anorexia Self Help, Inc., 120

California Colon Hygienists' Society, 104-105

Canadian Schizophrenia Foundation, 342-343

CANCER, 51-54

Cancer Control Society, 53-54

Cancer Research Institute, 55

CANDIDA ALBICANS, 66-67

Candida Research and Information Foundation, 66

Cardiac Alert, 178-179

Center for Frontier Sciences, 264-265

Center for Health Action, 479

Center for Medical Consumers, 239-240

Center for Traditional Acupuncture, 331

Cesareans/Support Education and Concern, 482-483

CFIDS Association, Inc., 99-100

CHELATION THERAPY, 68-70

CHILDBIRTH, 71-87

Childbirth Without Pain Education Association, 75-76

Child Health Alert, 90-91

Childhood, 373-374

CHILDHOOD AILMENTS, 88-98

Child Psychopharmacology Information Center, 91-92

Children With Attention Deficit Disorders, 92-93

Children's Hospice, International, 200

Choice, 247-248

Chronic Fatigue Immune Dysfunction Syndrome Society Int'l, 100-101

CHRONIC FATIGUE SYNDROME, 99-101

CIRCUMCISION, 102

Citizens for Alternative Health Care, 248-249

Coalition for Alternatives in Nutrition and Healthcare, Inc., 249-250

Co-Dependents Anonymous, 466-467

COLITIS AND CROHN'S DISEASE, 103

College of Optometrists in Vision Development, 143-144

COLON THERAPY, 104-105

COLOR THERAPY, 106

Committee for Truth In Psychiatry, 255-256

COMPUTER DATABASE SEARCHING, 107-108

Consciousness Village, 265

Consumers Advocating the Legalization of Midwifery, 76-77

Consumers United for Food Safety, 157-158

Cooking for Survival Consciousness, 392

Council for Responsible Nutrition, 393

Cranial Academy, 361

Crohn's & Colitis Foundation of America, Inc., 103

CRYSTAL HEALING, 109

Delicious, 394-395

DENTAL HEALTH, 110-114

Dinshah Health Society, 106

Dr. John W. Tintera Memorial Hypoglycemia Lay Group, 208-209

Doctor's People Newsletter, 240-241

Do It Now Foundation, 463-464

Durk Pearson & Sandy Shaw's *Life Extension Newsletter*, 231-232

DYSLEXIA AND SCOPTOPIC SENSITIVITY SYNDROME, 115-117

Earthwise Consumer, 128-129

EastWest, 221

EATING DISORDERS, 118-123

ECH_2O_2, Inc., 349

Edell Health Letter, 395-396

Ellon Bach USA, 150

ENDOMETRIOSIS, 124-125

Endometriosis Association, 124-125

Environmental Dental Association, 110-111

Environmental Health & Light Research Institute, Inc., 447-448

Environmental Health Network, 129-130

Environmental Health Watch, 131-132

ENVIRONMENTAL ILLNESS, 126-139

Environmental Nutrition, 396-397

Enviro-Tech Products, 49-50

EPILEPSY, 140-141

Epilepsy Foundation of America, 140-141

Exceptional Cancer Patients, 467-468

Exceptional Parent, 94

Executive Health Report, 397-398

EYE DISORDERS, 142-146

Federation of Straight Chiropractic Organizations, 362
Feingold Association of the United States, 95
Feldenkrais Guild, 362-363
Feldenkrais Resources, 363
FITNESS, 147-149
Flotation Tank Association, 460-461
FLOWER ESSENCE REMEDIES, 150-151
Flower Essence Services, 151
FOOD ALLERGIES, 152-156
FOOD IRRADIATION, 157-159
Forefront—Health Investigations, 232-233
Foundation for Advancement in Cancer Therapy, 56-57
Foundation for the Advancement of Innovative Medicine, 250-251
Foundation for Innovation in Medicine, 398-399
Foundation for Research of Natural Therapies, 2-3
Friends of Homebirth, 77-78

Gerson Institute, 57-58
G-Jo Institute, 332
Gluten Intolerance Group of North America, 154
Green Earth, 322-323
Greenkeeping, 132-133

HANDICAPPED, 160-161
HEAD INJURIES, 165-166
HEADACHES, 162-164
HEALING CENTERS, 167-168
Healing Currents, 399-400
Health and Energy Institute, 158-159
Health and Healing, 400-401
Health Consciousness, 402
Health Education AIDS Liaison, 4

Health Letter, 244-245
Health News & Review, 403
Health Resource, 170-171
HEALTH SELF-EDUCATION, 169-175
Health World, 16-17
Healthy Mothers, Healthy Babies, 78-79
HEARING PROBLEMS, 176-177
HEART DISEASE, HIGH BLOOD PRESSURE, AND STROKE, 178-183
Heart Disease Research Foundation, 179-180
Hellerwork, Inc., 364-365
Help Anorexia & Bulimia, Inc., 121
Help for Incontinent People, 214-215
HERBALISM, 184-191
Herb Research Foundation, 186
HERPES, 192-193
HERS Foundation, 483-484
Hippocrates Health Institute, 301-302
Holistic Dental Association, 111
Holistic Dental Digest, 112
Homeopathic Academy of Naturopathic Physicians, 195-196
Homeopathic Educational Services, 196-197
HOMEOPATHY, 194-199
HOPE Heart Institute, 180-181
HOSPICE, 200-201
Human Ecology Action League, 133-134
Huxley Institute for Biosocial Research, Inc., 344-345
HYPNOTHERAPY, 202-207
HYPOGLYCEMIA, 208-210
Hypoglycemia Association, Inc., 209-210

IMAGERY, 211-213
INCONTINENCE, 214-216

Independent Citizens Research Foundation for the Study of Degenerative Diseases, Inc., 251-252

Informed Homebirth/Informed Birth & Parenting, 79

Institute for Physical Fitness, 365-366

Institute for the Advancement of Health, 266-267

Institute for the Advancement of Human Behavior, 267-268

Institute for the Study of Human Knowledge, 268-269

Institute of Behavioral Kinesiology, 280-281

Institute of Noetic Sciences, 269-270

Internal Arts Magazine, 333-334

International Academy of Nutrition and Preventive Medicine, 404-405

International Academy of Oral Medicine and Toxicology, 113

International Association for Medical Assistance to Travelers, 476

International Association for Oxygen Therapy, 350

International Association of Cancer Victors and Friends, Inc., 58-59

International Association of Professional Natural Hygienists, 287

International Bio-Oxidative Medicine Foundation, 351-352

International Childbirth Education Association, 80-81

International Chiropractic Association, 366-367

International College of Applied Kinesiology, 281

International Dental Health Foundation, 114

International Forum on New Science, 270-271

International Foundation for Homeopathy, 197

International Foundation of Oriental Medicine, 334

International Health Federation, 67

International Institute for Bioenergetic Analysis, 271-272

International Institute of Reflexology, 335

International Journal of Aromatherapy, 32-33

International Journal of Biosocial and Medical Research, 302-303

International Medical and Dental Hypnotherapy Association, 206

International Myopia Prevention Association, 144-145

International School of Shiatsu, 336

International Society for the Study of Subtle Energies and Energy Medicine, 17-18

International Veterinary Acupuncture Society, 478-479

IRIDOLOGY, 217-218

Irlen Institute for Perceptual and Learning Development, 115-116

Jin Shin Do Foundation for Bodymind Acupressure, 337

John F. Kennedy University, 272

Journal of Alternative and Complementary Medicine, 19-20

Journal of Naturopathic Medicine, 291-292

Just Say No, International, 464-465

La Leche League International, 374-375

Lafayette University, 171-172

Let's Live, 405-406

Life Extension Foundation, 234-235

Life Science Institute, 287-288

Lifespan Associates, 109

LIFESTYLE, 219-227

Lifestyle Medicine Institute, 222-223

Linus Pauling Institute of Science and Medicine, 59-60, 181-182

Lloyd Library and Museum, 187

Longevity, 235-236

LONGEVITY AND AGING, 228-236

LUPUS ERYTHEMATOSIS, 237-238

Lupus Foundation of America, Inc., 237-238

Macrobiotics Today, 406-407

Maharishi Ayur-Veda Association of America, 44-45

Mastering Food Allergies, 155-156

McKenzie Institute, 367-368

MEDICAL CONSUMERISM, 239-244

MEDICAL/HEALTH CARE FRAUD, 244-245

MEDICAL/HEALTH CARE FREEDOM OF CHOICE, 246-254

MEDICAL/HEALTH CARE RIGHTS, 255-257

Medical Herbalism, 188

Meditation, 273-274

MEDLARS, 107

Melpomene Institute for Women's Health Research, 485

Midwives' Alliance of North America, 81-82

MIND–BODY CONNECTION, 258-279

Mothering, 375-376

MUSCLE TESTING AND DIAGNOSIS, 279-284

Myotherapy Institute of Utah, 461-462

NAPRALERT, 108

NAPSAC, 82-83

National Alliance for the Mentally Ill, 256-257

National Anorexic Aid Society, 122

National Association for Drama Therapy, 433

National Association for Holistic Aromatherapy, 33-34

National Association for Music Therapy, 433-434

National Association for Poetry Therapy, 434-435

National Association of Anorexia Nervosa and Associated Disorders, 123

National Association of Childbearing Centers, 83-84

National Association of Neuro-Linguistic Programming, Inc., 435-436

National Asthma Education Program, 37

National Center for Environmental Health Strategies, 135-136

National Center for Homeopathy, 198-199

National Center for Stuttering, 453-454

National Coalition Against the Misuse of Pesticides, 382-383

National Commission for the Certification of Acupuncturists, 338

National Committee for Prevention of Child Abuse, 96

National Council of Acupuncture Schools and Colleges, 339

National Eye Research Foundation, 146

National Foundation for Asthma, Inc., 38-39

National Foundation for the Chemically Hypersensitive, 136-137

National Handicapped Sports, 160

National Headache Foundation, 163-164

National Head Injury Foundation, Inc., 165-166

National Health Federation, 253

National Hospice Organization, 201

National Information Center for Children and Youth with Handicaps, 97

National Institute for the Clinical Application of Behavioral Medicine, 274-275

National Iridology Research Association, 217-218

National Jewish Center for Immunology and Respiratory Medicine, 444-445

National Network to Prevent Birth Defects, 84-85

National Neurofibromatosis Foundation, Inc., 293-294

National Organization of Circumcision Resource Centers, 102

National Organization for Rare Disorders, Inc., 442-443

National Organization for Seasonal Affective Disorder, 448-449

National Osteoporosis Foundation, 347-348

National Pesticide Telecommunications Network, 383-384

National Psoriasis Foundation, 419-420

National Self-Help Clearinghouse, 468-469

National Society of Hypnotherapists, 207

National Stuttering Project, 454-455

National Therapeutic Recreation Society, 436-437

National Wellness Institute, Inc., 223-224

National Women's Health Network, 486

Natural Food and Farming, 323-324

Natural Healing Newsletter, 303-304

Natural Health, 407-408

NATURAL HYGIENE, 285-289

Natural Hygiene, Inc., 289

Natural Lifestyle and Your Health, 408-409

Natural Living Newsletter, 409-410

Natural Resources Defense Council, 384-385

NATUROPATHY, 290-292

NEUROFIBROMATOSIS, 293-294

New Frontier, 275-276

New York Open Center, Inc., 224

North American Academy of Musculoskeletal Medicine, 368-369

North American Nutrition & Preventive Medicine Foundation, Inc., 304-305

North American Society of Teachers of the Alexander Technique, 369-370

North American Vegetarian Society, 305-306

Nurse Healers—Professional Association, Inc., 276-277

Nutrition Action Healthletter, 307

Nutrition and Cancer, 61

NUTRITION AND DIET, 295-318

Nutrition Education Association, Inc., 308

Nutrition for Optimal Health Association, Inc., 410-411

Nutrition Health Review, 411-412

Nutrition News, 309

Nutrition Report, 310-311

OBSESSIVE-COMPULSIVE DIS-
ORDERS, 319-321
Obsessive Compulsive Informa-
tion Center, 319-320
OCD Foundation, Inc., 320-321
Omega Institute for Holistic Stud-
ies, 225-226
ORGANIC FOOD, 322-327
Organic Network, 324
ORIENTAL HEALING AND EX-
ERCISE, 328-341
ORTHOMOLECULAR NUTRI-
TION AND THERAPY, 342-346
Orton Dyslexia Society, 116-117
OSTEOPOROSIS, 347-348
Overeaters Anonymous, 481
OXIDATIVE THERAPIES, 349-352

PAIN RELIEF, 353-372
Pan American Allergy Society, 8-9
PARENTING, 373-378
PARKINSON'S DISEASE, 379-380
Parkinson's Education Program,
379-380
Patient Advocates for Advanced
Cancer Treatments, Inc., 62
Patient Rights Legal Action Fund,
254
Pediatrics for Parents, 376-377
People Against Cancer, 63
People's Medical Society, 241
PESTICIDES, 381-385
Physician's Committee for Re-
sponsible Medicine, 311-312
Phyto-Pharmica Review, 189
Planetree Health Resource, 172-
173
Port Townsend Health Letter, 20-21
Positive Pregnancy & Parenting
Fitness, 85-86
Practical Allergy Research Foun-
dation, 98

PREVENTION, 386-418
Prevention, 412-413
Preventive Medical Update, 413-414
Preventive Medicine Update, 312-313
Price-Pottenger Nutrition Founda-
tion, 313-314
Princeton BioCenter, 345-346
Priority Parenting, 377-378
Proprioceptive Writing Center,
437-438
PSORIASIS, 419-420
PSYCHOLOGICAL HEALING,
421-441
Public Voice, 242

Radix Institute, 439
RARE DISEASES, 442-443
Read Natural Childbirth Founda-
tion, Inc., 86-87
RECNAC/Project, 64-65
Resonance, 50
RESPIRATORY ILLNESSES, 444-
445
Rheumatoid Disease Foundation,
35-36
Rolf Institute, 370-371

Safe Water Foundation, 480
SCLERODERMA, 446
Scleroderma Association, 446
SEASONAL AFFECTIVE DISOR-
DER, 447-449
Second Opinion, 243
Self Help for Hard of Hearing Peo-
ple, Inc., 176-177
Shen Systems, 340
Simon Foundation, 215-216
SJÖGREN'S SYNDROME, 450-451
Sjögren's Syndrome Foundation,
Inc., 450-451 ·
Society for the Advancement of
Travel for the Handicapped,
161

Society for the Study of Biochemical Intolerance, 137-138
Society of Prospective Medicine, 415
Solstice, 21-22, 315
Sounds True Catalogue, 440
Spectrum, 416
Speech Foundation of America, 455-456
SPEECH PROBLEMS, 452-456
SPORTS MEDICINE, 457-458
Sprout House, 325
Sproutletter, 326-327
STRESS REDUCTION, 459-462
Stroke Foundation, Inc., 182-183
SUBSTANCE ABUSE, 463-465
SUPPORT GROUPS, 466-470

T'ai Chi, 340
TEMPOROMANDIBULAR JOINT DISEASE, 471-472
Temporomandibular Joint Research Foundation, 471-472
Therapeutic Herbalism, 190-191
TINNITUS, 473
Today's Living, 417
Total Health, 226-227
Touch For Health Foundation, 283-284
TOURETTE SYNDROME, 474-475

Tourette Syndrome Association, Inc., 474-475
Townsend Letter for Doctors, 22-23
Trager Institute, 371-372
TRAVELING ABROAD, 476
Tree Farm Communications, 173-174

United States Water Fitness Association, Inc., 148-149

Vegetarian Resource Group, 316
Vegetarian Times, 317-318
VETERINARY HEALTH CARE, 477-479
Volunteer—The National Center, 469-470

Wary Canary, 138-139
WATER FLUORIDATION, 479-480
WEIGHT LOSS, 481
Whole Health Institute, 277-278
Women for Sobriety, 487
WOMEN'S HEALTH ISSUES, 482-487
World Research Foundation, 174-175

Yoga Journal, 341